CANE FIGHTING

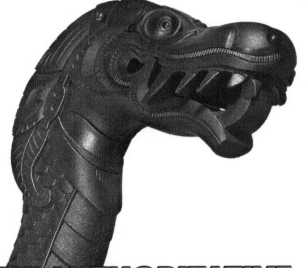

THE AUTHORITATIVE GUIDE TO USING THE CANE OR WALKING STICK FOR SELF-DEFENSE

SAMMY FRANCO

Also by Sammy Franco

Kubotan Power: Quick & Simple Steps to Mastering the Kubotan Keychain
The Heavy Bag Bible
The Widow Maker Compendium
Invincible: Mental Toughness Techniques for Peak Performance
Bruce Lee's 5 Methods of Attack
Unleash Hell: A Step-by-Step Guide to Devastating Widow Maker Combinations
Feral Fighting: Advanced Widow Maker Fighting Techniques
The Widow Maker Program: Extreme Self-Defense for Deadly Force Situations
Savage Street Fighting: Tactical Savagery as a Last Resort
Heavy Bag Workout
Heavy Bag Combinations
Heavy Bag Training
The Complete Body Opponent Bag Book
Stand and Deliver: A Street Warrior's Guide to Tactical Combat Stances
Maximum Damage: Hidden Secrets Behind Brutal Fighting Combinations
First Strike: End a Fight in Ten Seconds or Less!
The Bigger They Are, The Harder They Fall
Self-Defense Tips and Tricks
Gun Safety: For Home Defense and Concealed Carry
Out of the Cage: A Guide to Beating a Mixed Martial Artist on the Street
Warrior Wisdom: Inspiring Ideas from the World's Greatest Warriors
War Machine: How to Transform Yourself Into a Vicious and Deadly Street Fighter
1001 Street Fighting Secrets
When Seconds Count: Self-Defense for the Real World
Killer Instinct: Unarmed Combat for Street Survival
Street Lethal: Unarmed Urban Combat

Cane Fighting: The Authoritative Guide to Using the Cane or Walking Stick for Self-Defense
Copyright © 2016 by Sammy Franco
ISBN: 978-1-941845-30-1
Printed in the United States of America

Published by Contemporary Fighting Arts, LLC.
Visit us Online at: **SammyFranco.com**
Follow us on Twitter: **@RealSammyFranco**

For author interviews or publicity information, please send inquiries in care of the publisher.

II

Contents

"Speak softly and carry a big stick; you will go far."

– Theodore Roosevelt

Caution!

The author, publisher, and distributors of this book disclaim any liability from loss, injury, or damage, personal or otherwise, resulting from the information and procedures in this book. This book is for academic study only.

Remember, it's your sole responsibility to research and comply with all local, state and federal laws and regulations pertaining to the possession, carry, and use of a tactical cane or walking stick.

Before you begin any exercise or activity, including those suggested in this book, it is important to check with your physician to see if you have any condition that might be aggravated by strenuous training.

The information contained in this book is not designed to diagnose, treat, or manage any physical health conditions.

About Cane Fighting

Cane Fighting: The Authoritative Guide to Using the Cane or Walking Stick for Self-Defense is a practical book written for anyone who wants to learn how to use a cane or walking stick as a fighting weapon for real-world self-defense.

While seemingly inconspicuous, the cane or walking stick is a ubiquitous weapon for all ages, young and old, regardless of size or strength or experience and skill level. Most importantly, you don't need martial arts training to master this devastating self-defense weapon.

With over 200 photographs and step-by-step instructions, Cane Fighting is the authoritative resource for mastering the following weapons:

- **The Hooked Wooden Cane**
- **The Modern Tactical Combat Cane**
- **Walking Sticks**
- **The Irish Shillelagh**
- **The Bo Staff**

Unlike other books, Cane Fighting is devoid of tricky or flashy cane fighting moves that can get you injured or possibly killed when defending against a determined attacker. Instead, it arms you with practical and powerful cane fighting techniques that actually work in the chaos of real-life street assaults. In fact, the skills and techniques found in these pages are surprisingly simple and easy to apply.

Practitioners who regularly practice the skills and techniques featured in this book will establish a rock solid foundation for using the cane for personal defense. Moreover, the techniques featured in this book will significantly improve your overall self-defense skills, enhance your conditioning, and introduce you to a new and exciting method of personal protection.

Cane Fighting is based on my 30+ years of research, training and teaching the martial arts and combat sciences. In fact, I've taught these unique cane fighting skills to thousands of my students, and I'm confident they can help protect you and your loved ones during a time of need.

Cane Fighting has seven chapters, each one covering a critical aspect of training. Since this is both a skill-building workbook and training guide, feel free to write in the margins, underline passages, and dog-ear the pages.

Finally, I encourage you to read this book from beginning to end, chapter by chapter. Only after you have read the entire book should you treat it as a reference and skip around, reading those chapters that directly apply to you.

Good luck in your training!

- Sammy Franco

Chapter One
Choose Your Weapon Wisely

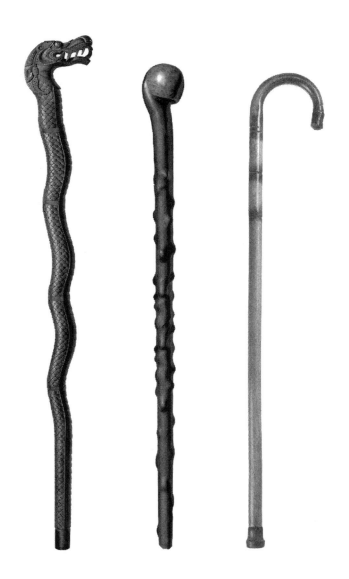

Before We Begin!

The purpose of this chapter is twofold. First, it will help you become familiar with the different features of the tactical cane. Second, it will help you choose the right stick for your self-defense needs.

Also, for reasons of simplicity, I'll be using the words "cane" and "walking stick" interchangeably throughout this book. Just remember, the self-defense techniques featured in this book can be readily applied with the cane, walking stick, Irish Shillelagh, and bo staff.

Why Carry a Cane for Self-Defense?

There are many advantages of using a tactical cane or walking stick for self-defense. First, it is an extremely effective impact tool that allows the average person to administer a devastating blow that far exceeds a typical punch. This fact is especially important for people who are either too small or weak to deliver fisted blows in a fight.

Second, unlike the gun or knife, the cane is ubiquitous tool that can be readily applied during an emergency self-defense situation. A casual stroll through the woods will certainly prove my point.

The walking stick is also versatile. It can be used as an intermediate use-of-force weapon that is useful in a wide variety of fighting environments and circumstances. However, the tactical cane can also be used during extreme self-defense situations, where deadly force is warranted and justified in the eyes of the law.

There are many other reasons why you should consider carrying a cane or walking stick for self-defense, here are a few more:

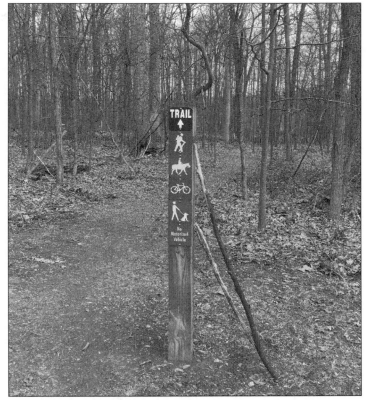

Canes and walking sticks are weapons of opportunity that are readily available.

- It's inconspicuous.

- It's lightweight.

- It's readily available.

- It makes a great everyday carry (EDC) item.

- It doesn't require reloading.

- It won't jam or misfire.

- It's legal to carry.

- It's an excellent impact weapon.

- It's both a lethal and non-lethal self-defense weapon.

Cane Fighting

- It permits a smaller or weaker person to generate tremendous striking power.

Regardless of your reasons for carrying a tactical cane or walking stick, remember it's your sole responsibility to research and comply with all local, state and federal laws and regulations pertaining to its possession, carry, and use.

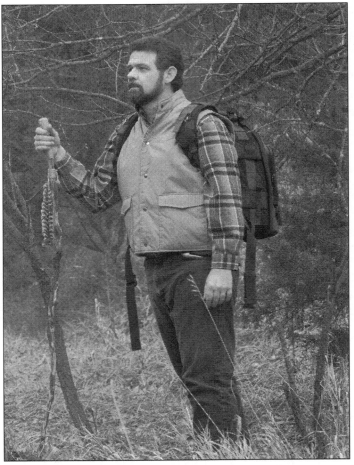

In the world of self-defense, the walking stick is a wolf in sheep's clothing. Does this man appear threatening?

No Two Canes are Alike!

There are hundreds, if not thousands, of different walking sticks on the market, however not all of them are suited for self-defense. In fact, some are downright awful. Choosing the right cane can make all the difference between surviving or dying in a high-risk self-defense altercation.

With so many different types of walking sticks on the market, it can be a bit overwhelming when trying to buy one for personal protection. For example, does it matter if it's made of high impact polypropylene or hardwood? Does it need to have a hook or a knob? Should I buy one that has a sharp point at its end? All of these questions can be answered by first understanding what components make a good tactical cane.

What is a Tactical Cane?

So exactly what is a *tactical cane* or *tactical walking stick* and why is it so important for personal protection. Essentially, a tactical cane is one that is specifically designed to handle the rigors of an

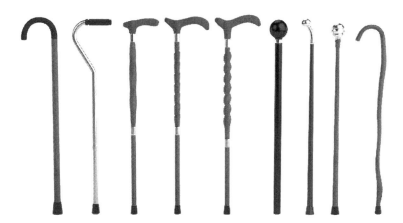

There are thousands of different canes and walking sticks available, however not all of them are designed for self-defense.

emergency self-defense situation. It should allow you to stop a criminal attacker dead in his tracks through the application of blunt force trauma. To accomplish this task, it must meet the following requirements.

- Sufficient length
- Appreciable weight
- Sufficient thickness
- Structural integrity
- Impact points
- Solid gripping
- Inconspicuous looking

Sufficient Length

For most people, the standard shaft length for a tactical cane is approximately 36 inches. However, you'll find that some walking sticks can be longer in length. In fact, some are as long as a bo staff. For our purposes, just be sure your cane or walking stick has a minimum length of 36 inches.

Appreciable Weight

If you intend on using your cane as a striking weapon, then it must have a minimum weight of approximately twenty ounces. Stick weight is important for one simple reason - striking power! Remember, your cane must have the capability to inflict immediate injury to your attacker.

Unfortunately, some commercial canes are made of lightweight aluminum, making them useless as self-defense weapons. Remember, you must have weight behind your cane strike. It must be hefty enough to incapacitate a large and powerful criminal attacker.

Sufficient Thickness

The shaft of your cane must also have a bit of thickness to it. Again, since its going to function as an impact weapon, it must it have a minimum circumference of 4.5 inches.

Structural Integrity

A tactical cane must be made of durable material that can withstand high impact. Avoid using canes that are made of hollow aluminum or light wood. Instead, find one that is constructed of either high impact polypropylene or hardwood.

Impact Points

Be sure your cane has impact points or ridges running down the shaft of the stick. This is important because it helps concentrate the force of your strike at the point of contact. A good example is Cold Steels Irish Blackthorn Shillelagh walking stick (figure right) which has clipped thorns on the shaft for both concentrated impact and weapon retention.

Solid Gripping

A tactical cane must have a solid gripping surface. Avoid using canes or walking sticks that have smooth polished shafts or high-gloss finishes, because they can become very slippery when your hands get wet from sweat, water, or blood.

Inconspicuous Looking

A tactical cane should also look harmless to the layperson. Remember, the last thing you want to do is bring attention to your weapon. Avoid carrying a cane that looks dangerous or threatening to other people. Avoid carrying one that have skulls, spikes, blades, sharp points, or any designs that look menacing.

Wooden Cane Nomenclature

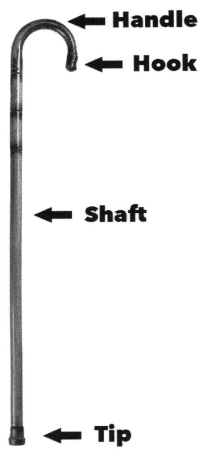

← **Handle**

← **Hook**

← **Shaft**

← **Tip**

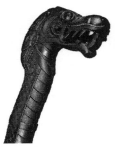

Contrary to popular belief, a tactical cane doesn't have to have a hooked wooden handle to be an effective self-defense weapon. In some cases, the hook can be a hindrance.

Tactical Cane Nomenclature

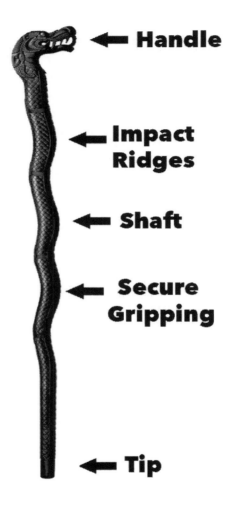

← **Handle**

← **Impact Ridges**

← **Shaft**

← **Secure Gripping**

← **Tip**

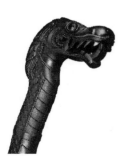

The primary function of a tactical cane and walking stick is to effectively strike your attacker. Therefore, it must have substantial weight and thickness to be a reliable impact weapon.

What About The Hook?

Despite what some people might say, you don't need a hook on your cane for it to be effective for personal defense. In fact, the hook portion of the cane is more of a novelty than anything else. Worst of all, it can be a big liability during a self-defense situation. Let me explain.

One of the most important concerns when using a cane for self-defense is weapon retention. In other words, it's essential for you to maintain control of your weapon at all times. Remember, if you attacker gets hold of your cane for even a second, it could be lights out for you.

Hooking, trapping or pinning your opponent's arms, groin, or legs with the hook of the cane can often result in a struggle with him. Moreover, attempting to leverage your opponent's limbs with your cane will likely result in him grabbing hold of your weapon and wrestling it away from you. This is especially true for smaller and weaker people who don't have the physical strength or endurance to engage in a tug of war match with their attacker. Fortunately, you can still use a hooked wooden cane for self-defense, just don't use the hook to ensnare your adversary.

The true combat utility of any tactical cane is to stop your attacker dead in his tracks through the application of blunt force trauma to specific vulnerable targets. It's that plain and simple!

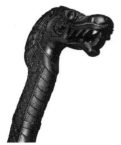

Since Cold Steel Inc. makes some of the best modern tactical canes for personal protection, we will be featuring them throughout this book. You can learn more by visiting their website at: coldsteel.com

The Irish Shillelagh

The truth is some of the best combat canes and walking sticks don't even have a hook. Take, for example, the Irish Shillelagh or blackthorn stick that is most often associated with Irish stick fighting.

This stout black stick has a large knob at the top that can easily cleave bone and split open a human skull. In fact, some Shillelaghs have their knobs hollowed out and then filled with molten lead to increase the striking force of the stick. Please believe me when I say that you never want to be at the wrong end of this stick!

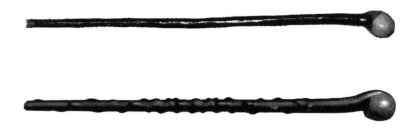

The Irish club or Shillelagh is both a wicked fighting tool and stylish walking stick, capable of inflicting tremendous damage. Pictured top, a traditional Irish Shillelagh. Pictured bottom, Cold Steel's modern interpretation of the Irish Blackthorn Shillelagh. Both are considered excellent tactical walking sticks.

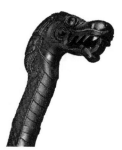

Shillelaghs are usually made from knotty blackthorn wood or oak because they are dense and heavy and less likely to crack during combat.

Cane Fighting

Chapter Two
Handling Your Weapon

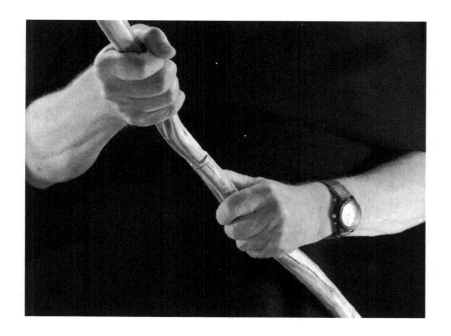

Cane Fighting Hand Grips

To effectively use a tactical cane or walking stick during an emergency self-defense situation, you're going to need to know about hand grips. Hand grips are vital because they determine which cane techniques you can apply and which targets you can strike.

For example, if you were holding your cane with a low point grip, it would be difficult and awkward to jab your adversary in his eyes. The grip is more suited for a diagonal strike to the opponent's temple or collarbone.

The Five Different Hand Grips

There are five grips that you should be familiar with, and they include:

- **One Hand grip**
- **High Point grip (one hand high, one low)**
- **Mid Point grip (one hand mid and one low)**
- **Low Point grip (two hands are low) (aka end grip)**
- **Quarterstaff grip**

One Hand Grip

The one hand grip is a natural looking position that is often used for everyday carry. This hand grip is also effective for both fist loading and quick wrist snapping techniques (more will be discussed).

However, let me offer one caveat. While the one hand grip does permit deceptive first strike capabilities, it should not be used when delivering a series of full-force power strikes. In fact, 95% of the cane strikes featured in this book should be performed with two hands. More will be explained in Chapter 5.

To perform the one hand grip, grasp the center of the walking stick so the exposed area of the weapon is equally above the thumb and below your pinky.

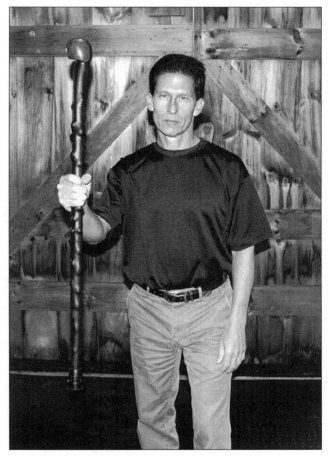

Pictured here, the one hand grip.

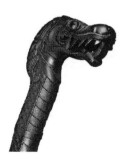

Hand grips need to be instinctual. Practice assuming the different grips everyday until all of them become second nature to you.

Fist Loading with the Cane

One of the hidden advantages of the one hand cane grip is "fist loading." This is the process of delivering fisted blows with the cane or walking stick placed in your hand. The fist loading concept is similar to punching someone with a roll of quarters in your fist. The added weight of the stick significantly increases the power of your punch. The following photographs demonstrate the fist loading principle.

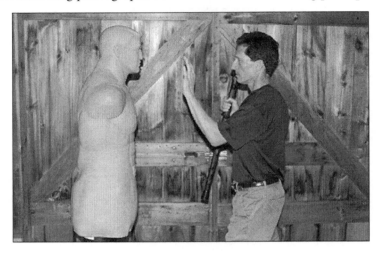

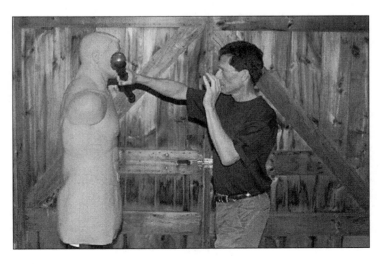

Wrist Snapping with the Cane

"Wrist snapping" is another skill performed with a one hand cane grip. This first strike technique allows you to hit your adversary with a quick snap of your wrist. However, to perform this action, you must have strong wrists and forearms. The following photographs demonstrate the wrist snapping principle.

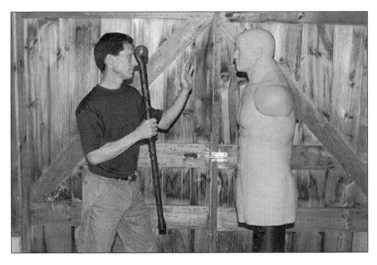

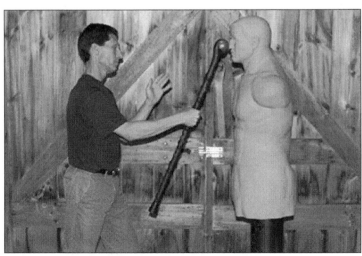

High Point Grip

The high point grip is used for both offensive and defensive purposes. To perform this two hand grip, grasp the cane with both of your hands, with one hand facing up and the other facing down, Both of your elbows should be slightly bent.

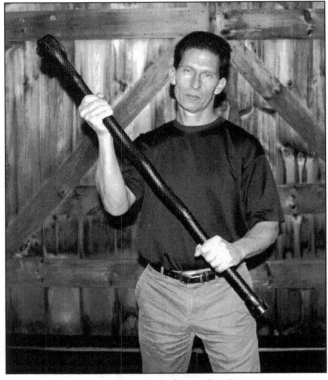

Pictured here, the high point hand grip.

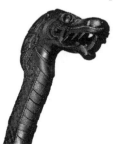

The high point grip is also ideal for performing cane deflection techniques. See chapter 6 for more information.

Mid Point Grip

The mid point grip is similar to the high point, except your top hand is placed in the middle portion of the cane. It's similar to holding and axe. Again, be sure both of your elbows are slightly bent.

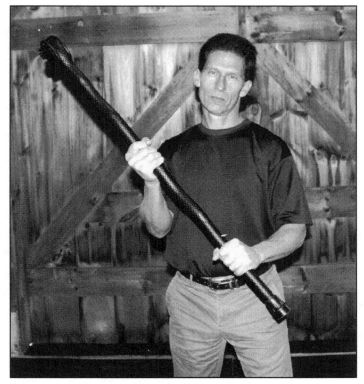

Pictured here, the mid point hand grip.

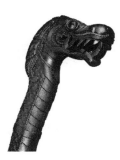

The mid point hand grip is perfect for delivering downward chopping strikes.

Low Point Grip

The low point hand grip is a power grip that permits you to swing the weapon with a tremendous amount of force. To assume this hand position, place both of your hands at the lower end of the walking stick, much like holding a big sword.

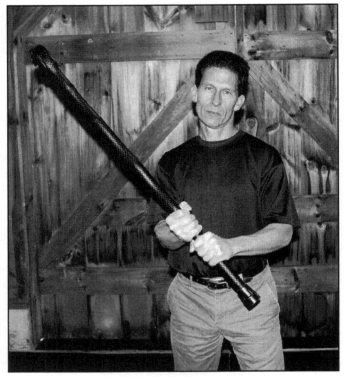

Pictured here, the low point hand grip.

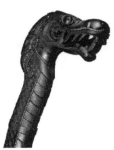

The low point hand grip is also called the baseball bat grip and end grip.

Quarterstaff Grip

The quarterstaff grip is similar to high point grip, except both of your hands are facing down. Again, make certain both of your hands are spaced equally apart from each other, with both of your elbows slightly bent.

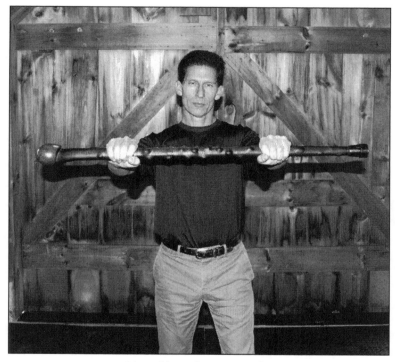

Pictured here, the quarterstaff grip.

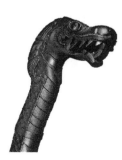

While the quarterstaff grip can be used for offensive applications, it's best used for blocking techniques.

Cane Fighting

Chapter Three
Stances and Concealment

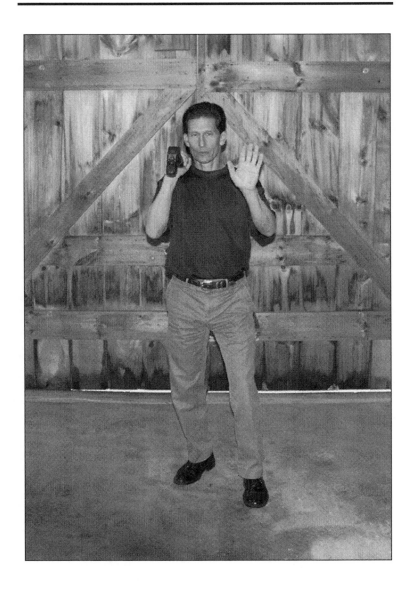

The Two Stages of Self-Defense

The stance is one of the most important and often neglected aspects of cane self-defense. However, before we can discuss the strategic implications of stances and weapon concealment, it's important to consider the two stages of self-defense and how they relate to cane fighting. Essentially, the two stages or phases of self-defense are:

- **Precontact Stage**
- **Contact Stage**

The Precontact Stage of Self-Defense

The precontact stage of self-defense refers to the moments before you physically engaging with your assailant. During the this stage of the conflict, you are either *aware* or *unaware* of the threat that awaits you.

The Aware State

During the aware state of the precontact phase, you have time (perhaps just a few seconds) to prepare yourself both mentally and physically for violence. In some cases, you might have the opportunity to engage in dialogue with your adversary before the situation leads to violence.

For example, let's say you are enjoying the night out with a few friends at a local bar. The place is dark, noisy and crowded which causes you to spill your drink on an inebriated patron. He immediately becomes enraged and begins to threaten you. You are experiencing an aware state of a precontact self-defense situation, requiring you to (hopefully) defuse the hostile person.

The Unaware State

During the unaware state of the precontact stage, you don't have

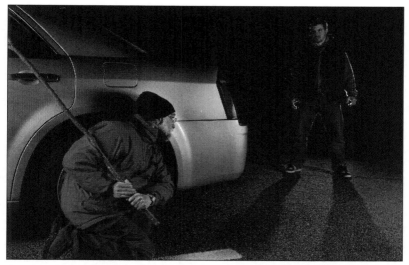

Awareness can make all the different during the precontact stage of self-defense. In this photo, the man on the left prepares to defend against his attacker.

time to prepare yourself mentally and physically for violence. In the moments before an attack, you're unaware of your adversary's presence. Essentially, you're caught off guard and never see the danger coming you way.

The best way to avoid such a situation is to try and work on your situational awareness skills. Situational awareness is total alertness, presence, and focus on virtually everything in your immediate surroundings.

With practice, you can train your senses to detect and assess the people, places, objects, and actions that can pose a danger to you

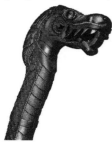

Very few people have refined their situational awareness skills. The reasons are many. Some are in denial about the prevalence of violent crime while others are too distracted by life's everyday pressures to pay attention to the hidden dangers that lurk around them. Whatever the reasons, poor awareness skills can get you into serious trouble.

and your loved ones. Do not think of situational awareness simply in terms of the five traditional senses of sight, sound, smell, taste, and touch. In addition, the very real powers of instinct and intuition must also be developed and eventually relied upon.

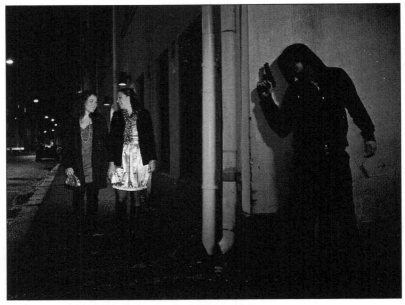

There is no denying the fact that poor awareness skills can get you into serious trouble.

Two vagrants congregating on the street corner or by your car, the stranger lingering at the mailboxes in your lobby, the delivery man at the door, a deserted parking lot, an alleyway near a familiar

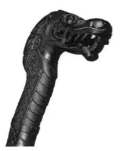

Seasoned criminal aggressors are looking for easy strikes - what they call the "vic." Barroom brawlers, street thugs, and muggers operate in the same basic manner. They look for the weak, timid, disoriented, and unaware victims.

sidewalk, a large limb hanging precariously from a tree . . . these are all obvious examples of persons, places, and objects that pose a threat to you. Situational awareness need not - and should not - be limited to preconceived notions about obvious sources of danger.

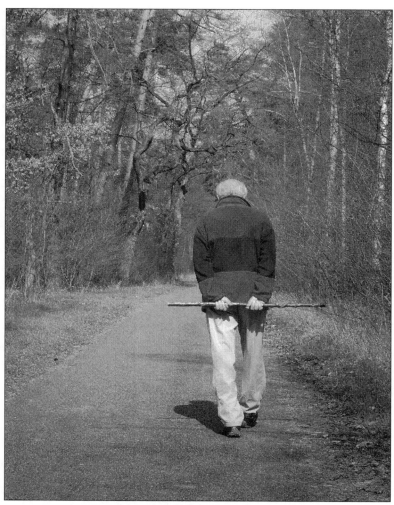

Situational awareness is total alertness, presence, and focus on virtually every-thing in your immediate surroundings. How would you rate this man's level of awareness?

The Contact Stage of Self-Defense

During the contact stage of self-defense, you are fighting with your assailant. For example, while attempting to de-escalate a drunk at the bar, he takes a swing at your head. You respond by blocking his attack and gaining control over the man.

Here's another example, you're on your way home from work and happen to walk past a dark alleyway. When you turn the corner, a stranger grabs you from behind and places you in a rear bear hug. You immediately react by breaking free from the hold and counter striking. The assailant falls to the ground, allowing you to safely escape from the scene.

As you can see, both contact stage examples require you to react to the threat to ensure your survival.

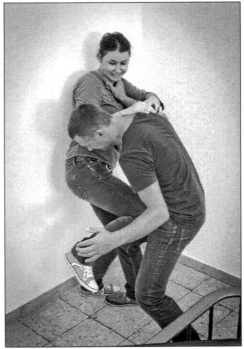

Pictured here, a woman fights back during the contact stage of self-defense.

Cane Combat and the Self-Defense Stages

I have some good news! The cane and walking stick can be used during both the precontact and contact stages of self-defense. Let's first talk about using it during the precontact stage.

Cane Applications During the Precontact Stage

Using the cane during the precontact stage will require you to *partially conceal* it from your potential adversary. As you already know, both the cane and walking stick are long objects that are difficult to hide from your attacker. However, in this chapter, I'm going to teach you some effective ways to help obscure the weapon.

Partially concealing your weapon is important for some of the following reasons:

- **Escalation Prevention** - As I mentioned earlier, in the precontact stage of self-defense, there might be an opportunity for you to try and de-escalate or diffuse a hostile person from using violence. In such a scenario, you want your cane at the ready, but you don't want to advertise its presence. Doing so might escalate the situation.

- **The Element of Surprise** - There's an old saying, "The hardest punch, is the one you never see coming." The same adage applies to cane fighting. If possible, don't let the adversary know you have a weapon. You want the element of surprise if and when you decide to fight back.

Obscuring your cane during the precontact stage of self-defense will require you to master two critical, yet strategic postures: the high and low concealment stances. Let's take a look at each one.

The High Concealment Cane Stance

The first stance I am going to teach you is the high concealment stance, and it is used when you are faced with a precontact self-defense situation.

This stance requires you to conceal your cane over your shoulder, with the tip, knob or handle pointing directly at your adversary. The high concealment stance is an ideal posture because it provides you with the following benefits:

- **Partial concealment**
- **Speed of deployment**
- **Striking power**
- **Mobility**
- **Balance and Stability**
- **Offensive fluidity**
- **Maximizes weapon reach**

The key to this deceptive cane fighting stance is the centerline. The centerline is an imaginary vertical line that divides your body in half. Located on this line are some of your vital targets (i.e., eyes, nose, chin, throat, solar plexus, and groin).

When confronted by a threatening adversary, it's important to position your centerline approximately forty-five degrees from the opponent. This will help protect your vital targets and help provide stability to your stance.

How to Assume the Stance

To assume the high concealment stance, stand with both of your legs approximately shoulder width apart. Position your body at a forty-five degree angle from the adversary. Keep your knees bent,

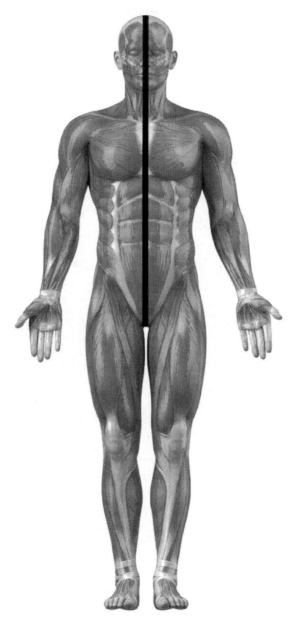

The stances featured in this book are predicated on the centerline.

Cane Fighting

both hands up, and fifty percent of your weight on each leg. And remember to keep your neck, shoulders, and arms relaxed.

Next, keep both of your hands up (one holding the cane and the other with your palm facing the adversary). You can hold your cane with either the tip, handle or knob facing the opponent.

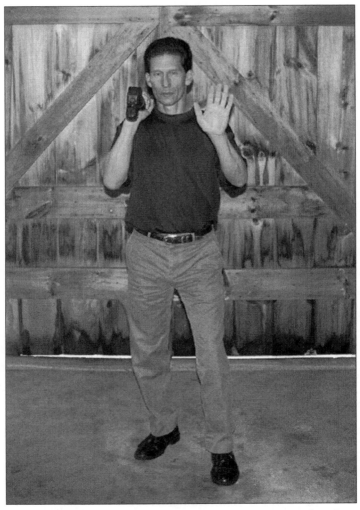

Pictured here, front view of the high concealment stance. Notice how the length of the weapon is partially concealed.

To prevent displaying the full-length of the cane to the assailant, remember to keep the stick pointing straight at him. Your goal is to minimize the presence of the weapon. Most importantly, obscuring the cane in this fashion provides you with the element of surprise, if and when you have to deploy it.

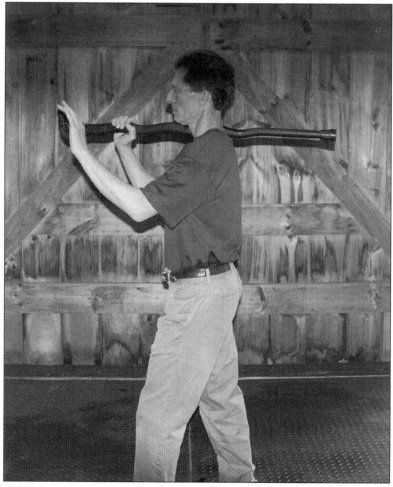

Side view of the high concealment stance.

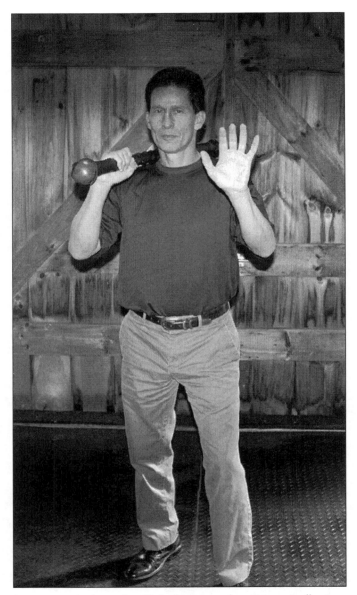

A common mistake made with the high concealment stance is allowing the cane to point sideways, giving the adversary a good view of the weapon.

Striking First During the Encounter

One of the greatest advantages of the high concealment stance is that it offers you the ability to strike your assailant first during the threatening encounter.

Whenever you are face-to-face with a criminal assailant, and there is no way to escape the threat of physical assault, you must take the initiative and strike first, strike fast, strike with authority, and keep the pressure on.

This reaction is called the first-strike principle, and it is essential to the process of neutralizing a vicious criminal. Keep in mind that if you wait for the assailant to strike you first, he might injure or kill you or force you into an irreversible defensive position that prevents you from issuing an effective counterstrike.

My first-strike principle is also important because it uses the element of surprise and thereby reduces your chances of injury by quickly putting an end to your dangerous encounter. For example, a quick and powerful downward cane strike to the attacker's collarbone can immediately take him out of commission.

Of course, you must also concern yourself with the law. You must be certain that your initial attack is warranted and justified in the eyes of the law. Therefore, it's essential to assess the threatening situation accurately and choose the appropriate self-defense response.

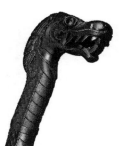

If you would like to learn more about the First Strike principle, see my book First Strike: End a Fight in Ten Seconds or Less.

Striking From The High Concealment Stance

The following photo sequence demonstrates just how easy it is to initiate a first strike from the high concealment stance.

Step 1: Start by facing the adversary in a high concealment stance. Be certain your stance appears natural and nonthreatening.

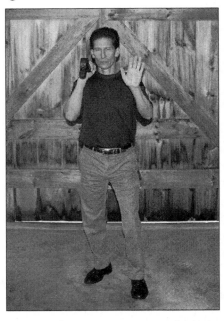

Step 2: Next, with your free hand, reach across your chest and grab the cane in a low point grip.

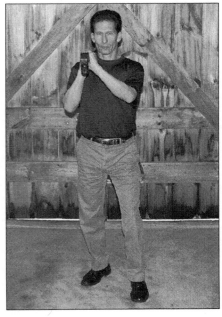

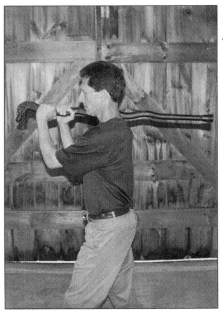

Pictured here, a side view of the low point grip

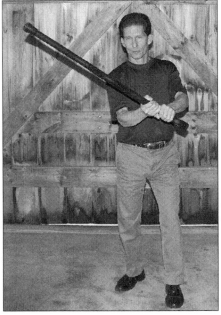

Step 3: Swing you cane diagonally downward at your opponent.

The Low Concealment Cane Stance

The low concealment stance is used when your cane is low to the ground, and you're confronted with a *potential* threat.

Consider, for example, standing on a street corner waiting for a taxi, when suddenly you are approached by someone asking for directions. In this situation, you're uncertain if the stranger is innocently asking for assistance or if he's setting you up for an attack. Nevertheless, it's important to utilize a concealment technique in the event the stranger has nefarious intentions.

The low concealment stance is ideal because it obscures your cane behind your leg, yet it permits rapid offensive deployment (if necessary).

Distance Matters!

Since the low concealment stance requires one of your hands to drop to your side, it should only be used when the adversary is at the neutral zone.

The neutral zone is the distance where the adversary is too far away from you to strike with his limbs. The strategic implication of the neutral zone is that it creates precious distance between you and your adversary. This, in turn, allows you to assess your situation and choose the appropriate tactical response.

However, if your adversary attacks you first, the neutral zone

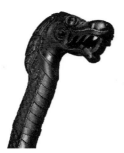

Proximity is a vital consideration in both armed and unarmed combat. The farther away you are from an assailant, the greater your defensive reaction time, and the greater the visual picture you will have of your emergency situation. The closer you are to your assailant, the fewer options you have.

also provides you with necessary reaction time to adequately protect yourself. Beware, however, because not all assailants, self-defense situations, or environments will a afford you the luxury of maintaining a neutral zone.

How to Assume the Stance

Like the high concealment posture, the low concealment stance also requires you to partially conceal your weapon from the adversary. The only difference is your cane is touching the floor and therefore must be obscured by your legs.

To assume the low concealment stance, keep your feet approximately shoulder width apart. Angle your body approximately forty-five degrees from your adversary with both of your knees slightly bent. Keep fifty percent of your weight distributed over each leg and remain relaxed and prepared.

Next, place your cane against the side of your thigh, with the weapon being partially concealed behind your rear leg. If time permits, keep your free hand up with your palm facing the opponent. Remember that your stance must always appear natural and nonthreatening to the adversary.

Like the other stance, the low concealment stance also allows you to effectively launch a first strike at your adversary. Again, be certain your actions and legally and morally justified in the eyes of the law.

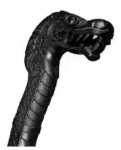

In order for the low concealment stance to work effectively, you must appear natural and nonthreatening to the adversary.

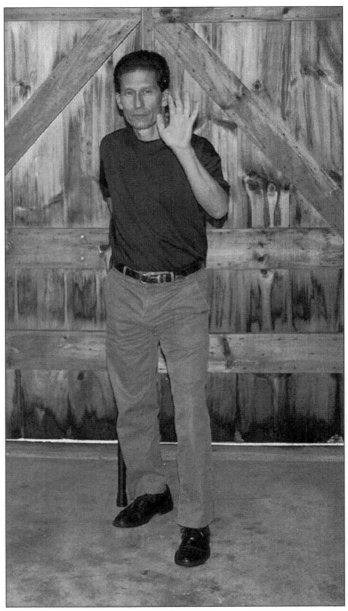

Pictured here, front view of the low concealment stance.

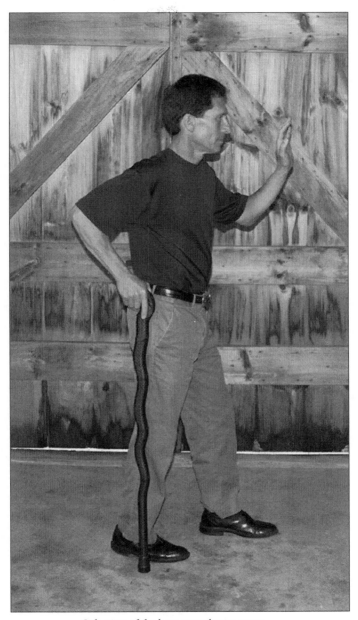

Side view of the low concealment stance.

Striking From The Low Concealment Stance

The following photo sequence demonstrates the efficiency of initiating a first strike from a low concealment stance.

Step 1: Start by facing the adversary in a low concealment posture. Remember, your stance must always appear natural and nonthreatening to the opponent.

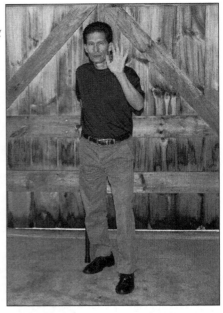

Step 2: Next, simultaneously join both of your hands together in a low point grip, and swing your cane at your attacker.

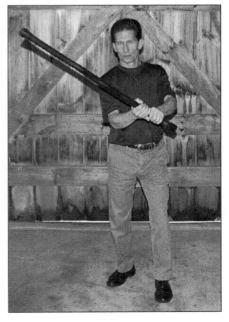

Chapter Four
Target Areas

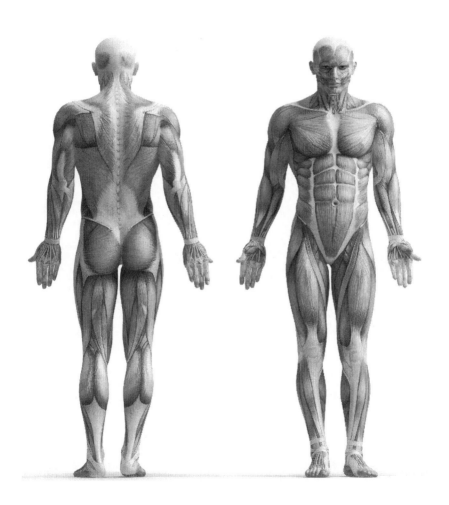

What is Target Awareness?

Defending yourself with a walking stick requires you to possess a variety of fighting attributes. Essentially, attributes are mental and physical qualities that enhance your combat skills and techniques. Some attributes include power, speed, accuracy, timing, and balance.

However, when it comes to cane fighting, one of the most important attributes is target awareness. Simply put, target awareness is a culmination of five interdependent principles. They are:

- Target orientation
- Target recognition
- Target selection
- Target impaction
- Target exploitation

Let's first take a look at target orientation and see how it directly relates to the cane.

Target Orientation

Target orientation means having a workable knowledge of specific anatomical targets that are especially vulnerable to attack. These targets can be found in one of three possible target zones.

Target Zones

Zone 1 (head region) - includes targets related to the assailant's senses, including the eyes, temples, nose, chin, and back of neck.

Zone 2 (neck, torso, and groin) - includes targets related to the assailant's breathing, including the throat, solar plexus, ribs, and groin.

Zone 3 (legs and feet) - includes targets related to the assailant's mobility, including the thighs, knees, shins, and instep/toes.

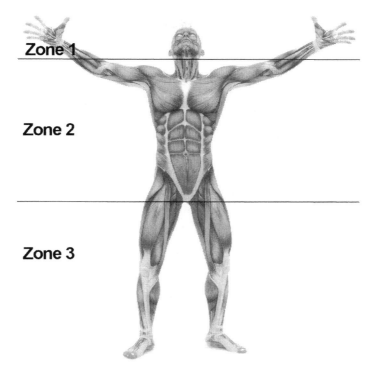

Simply knowing the specific locations of various anatomical targets is not enough. Target orientation also requires that you have a strong understanding of the medical implications of striking these targets.

As a matter of fact, if you intend on using a tactical cane for personal defense, you have a moral and legal responsibility to know the medical implications of each and every offensive strike and technique.

A responsible law abiding citizen must know exactly which anatomical targets will stun, incapacitate, disfigure, maim, or kill the adversary. Therefore, let's take a closer look at these targets and the medical implications of each one.

Cane Fighting Targets

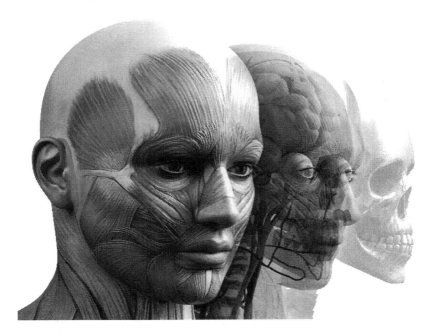

The best targets for cane fighting are bony surfaces of the body that are only protected by a thin layer of skin or soft tissue. Luckily, the human body has several anatomical targets that are especially vulnerable to cane strikes. Let's take a look at the viable targets.

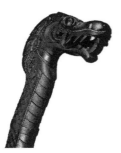

Cane fighting is a science requiring precise targeting. Randomly striking at your adversary will often yield poor results and will most certainly enrage him.

Eyes

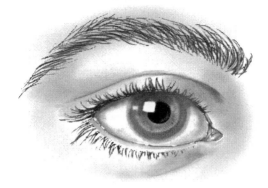

The eyes are ideal targets for a good target because they are extremely sensitive and difficult to protect. The eyes can be poked, raked, and gouged with both the handle and tip of your cane.

Depending on the force of your strike, it can cause numerous injuries, including watering of the eyes, hemorrhaging, blurred vision, temporary or permanent blindness, severe pain, rupture, shock, and even unconsciousness.

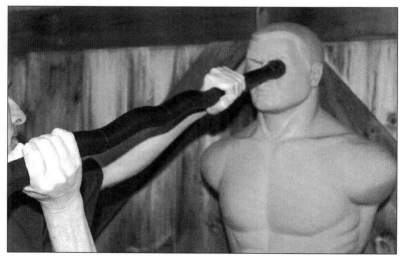

In this photo, the practitioner delivers a jab to the eyes with the tip of the cane.

Temple

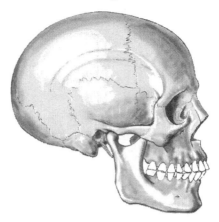

The temple or sphenoid bone is a thin, weak bone located on both sides of the skull approximately one inch from the assailant's eye. Because of its inherently weak structure and close proximity to the brain, a very powerful cane strike to this anatomical target can be deadly. Other possible injuries include unconsciousness, hemorrhaging, concussion, shock, and coma.

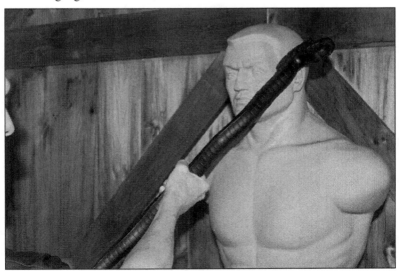

Striking the temple with the handle of the cane.

Nose

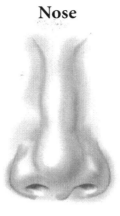

The nose is made up of a thin bone, cartilage, numerous blood vessels, and many nerves. It is a particularly good impact target because it stands out from the assailant's face and can be struck in three different directions (up, straight, down). A moderate blow can cause stunning pain, eye-watering, temporary blindness, and hemorrhaging. A powerful cane strike can result in shock and unconsciousness.

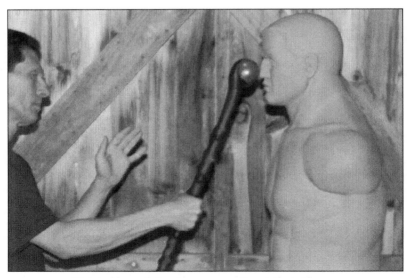

Pictured here, delivering a preemptive strike to the nose.

Chin

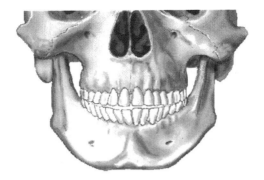

The chin is also a good striking target. When the chin is struck at a 45-degree angle, shock waves are transmitted to the cerebellum and cerebral hemispheres of the brain, resulting in paralysis and immediate unconsciousness.

Depending on the force of your blow, other possible injuries include broken jaw, concussion, and whiplash to the assailant's neck.

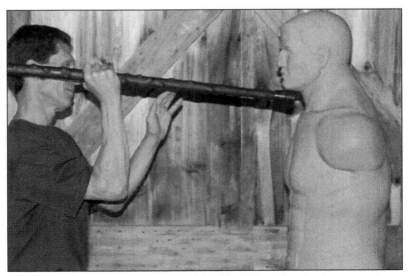

In this photo, a preemptive strike delivered to the chin.

Back of Neck

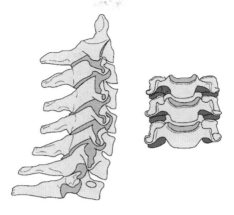

The back of the neck consists of the first seven vertebrae of the spinal column. They function as a circuit board for nerve impulses from the brain to the body. The back of the neck is a lethal target because the vertebrae are poorly protected. A very powerful cane strike to the back of the assailant's neck can cause shock, unconsciousness, a broken neck, complete paralysis, coma, and dea

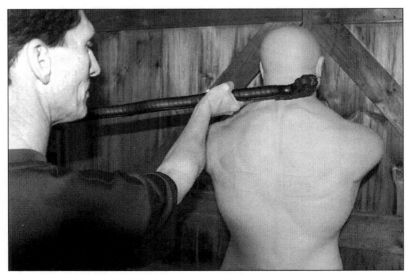

Striking the back of the neck should only be done in life and death situations.

Spine

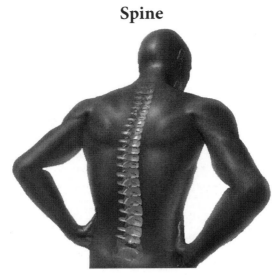

Like the back of the neck, the spine also functions as a circuit board for nerve impulses from the brain to the body. A powerful strike to the assailant's spine can cause shock, unconsciousness, complete paralysis, coma, and death.

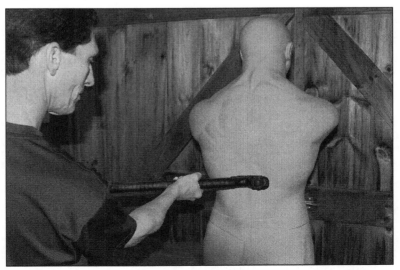

Like the back of the neck, the spine should only be struck in life and death self-defense situations.

Throat

The throat is considered a lethal target because it is only protected by a thin layer of skin. This region consists of the thyroid, hyaline, cricoid cartilage, trachea, and larynx. The trachea, or windpipe, is a cartilaginous cylindrical tube that measure four and a half inches in length and approximately one inch in diameter.

A direct and powerful cane strike to this target may result in unconsciousness, blood drowning, massive hemorrhaging, strangulation, and death. If the thyroid cartilage is crushed, hemorrhaging will occur, the windpipe will quickly swell shut, and the assailant will die of suffocation.

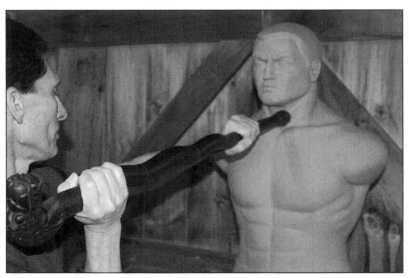

Striking the throat can also be deadly.

Collarbone

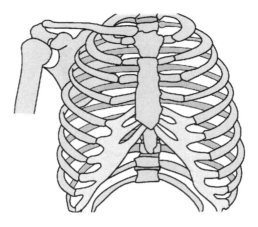

While the collar bone is not an ideal target for unarmed fighting, it's a great target for a cane strike. As a matter of fact, forcefully striking the collar bone with a walking stick can easily break it, resulting in extreme pain and difficulty moving the affected arm.

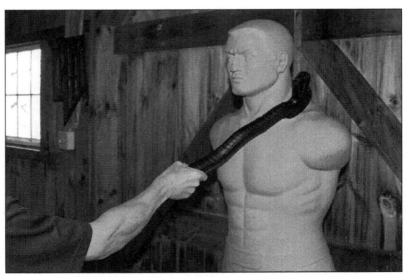

Striking the collarbone with the handle of the cane.

Ribs

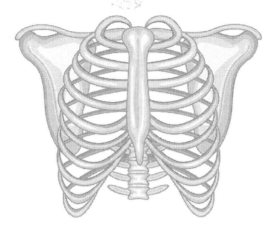

A moderate cane strike to the anterior region of the ribs may cause severe pain and shortness of breath. An extremely powerful 45-degree blow could break the assailant's rib and force it into a lung, resulting in the lung's collapse, internal hemorrhaging, air starvation, unconsciousness, excruciating pain, and possible death.

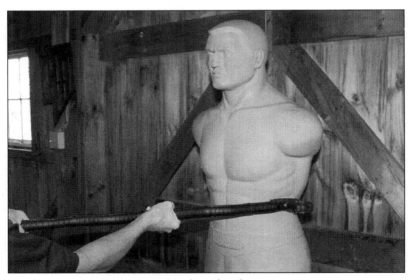

Attacking the ribs.

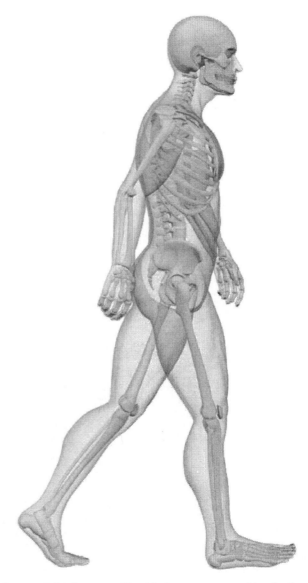

The human skeletal system offers ideal target opportunities for the cane.
Attacking the skeletal system produces immediate results!

Solar Plexus

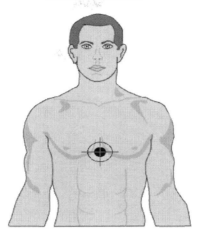

The solar plexus is a large collection of nerves situated below the sternum in the upper abdomen. A moderate blow to this area can cause nausea, pain, and shock, making it difficult for the adversary to breathe properly. A powerful cane strike to the solar plexus can result in severe abdominal pain and cramping, air starvation, and shock.

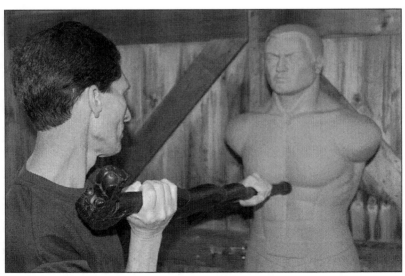

Attacking the solar plexus with the tip of the cane.

Groin

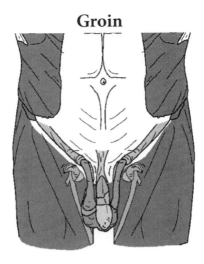

A moderate cane strike to an assailant's groin can cause a variety of possible reactions, including severe pain, nausea, vomiting, shortness of breath, and possible sterility. A powerful strike to the groin may crush the scrotum and the testes against the pubic bones, causing shock and unconsciousness.

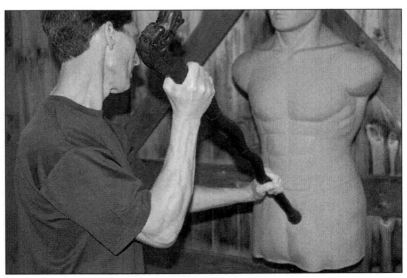

Attacking the groin with a downward thrust.

Thighs

Although you can strike the leg at a variety of different angles, the ideal location is the assailant's common peroneal nerve located on the side of the thigh, approximately four inches above the knee. Striking this area can result in extreme pain and immediate immobility of the afflicted leg. An extremely hard cane strike to the thigh may result in a fracture of the femur, internal bleeding, severe pain, intense cramping, and long-term immobility.

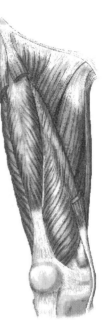

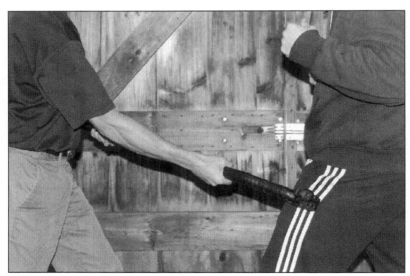

Striking the thigh with the handle of the cane.

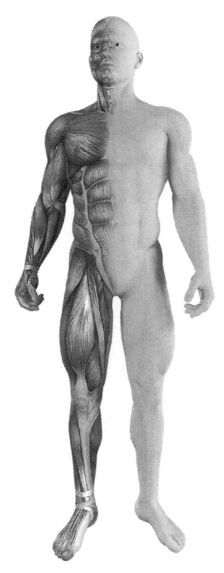

When striking your adversary with the walking stick, remember to aim for bony targets that are only protected by a thin layer of skin. Avoid striking muscular parts of the body.

Knees

The knees are relatively weak joints that are held together by a number of supporting ligaments. When the assailant's leg is locked or fixed in position and a forceful strike is delivered to the front of the joint, the crucial ligaments will tear, resulting in excruciating pain, swelling, and immobility.

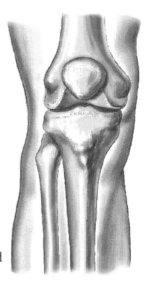

Located on the front of the knee joint is the kneecap, or patella, which is made of a small, loose piece of bone. The patella is also vulnerable to possible dislocation by a direct, forceful hit. Severe pain, swelling, and immobility may also result.

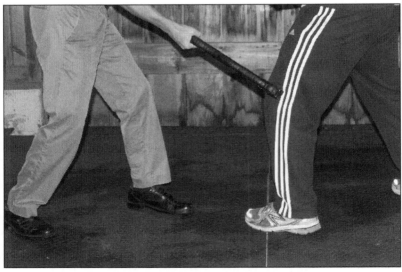

Attacking the knee with the handle of the cane.

Shins

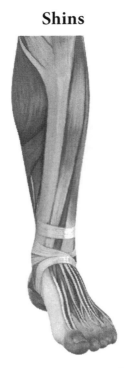

The shins are also very sensitive targets because they are only protected by a thin layer of skin. A powerful blow delivered to this target may fracture it easily, resulting in extreme pain, hemorrhaging, and immobility of the afflicted leg.

Elbows

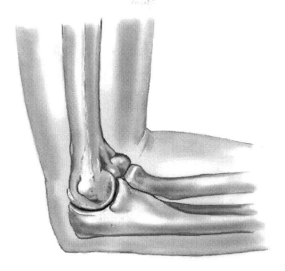

Because the elbows are only protected by a thin layer of skin, they are also ideal targets for cane strikes. In fact, striking the elbow with a moderate amount of force can lead to immediate paralysis of the limb.

Fingers and Hands

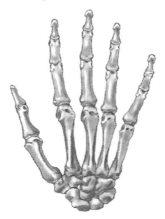

The fingers and hands are exceptionally weak and vulnerable and make ideal cane striking targets. The fingers can easily be jammed, sprained, broken, and torn. While a broken hand might not stop a determined attacker, it will certainly prevent him from delivering a fisted blow.

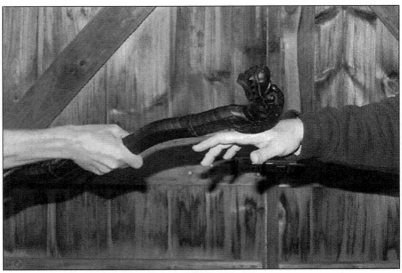

Striking the hand with the handle of the cane.

Understanding Use-of-Force

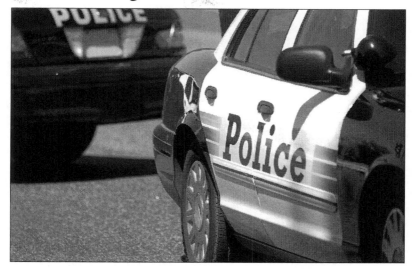

One of the most difficult aspects of using a cane in a self-defense situation is determining exactly how much force can be applied. Well, since every personal defense situation is unique, there is no simple answer.

First, you must never use force against another person unless it is absolutely justified in the eyes of the law. Basically, use-of-force is broken down into two levels: lethal and nonlethal.

Lethal force is defined as the amount of force that can cause serious bodily injury or death. Nonlethal force is an amount of force that does not cause serious bodily injury or death.

Keep in mind that any time you use physical force against another person, you run the risk of having a civil suit filed against you. Remember, anyone can hire a lawyer and file a suit for damages. Likewise, anyone can file a criminal complaint against you. Whether criminal charges will be brought against you depends upon the prosecutor's or grand jury's view of the facts.

Cane Fighting

Second, a cane or walking stick should only be used as an act of protection against unlawful injury or the immediate risk of unlawful injury. If you decide to strike your adversary, you'd better be certain that a reasonable threat exists and that it is absolutely necessary to protect yourself from immediate danger. Remember, the decision to use a self-defense weapon must always be a last resort, after all other means of avoiding violence have been exhausted.

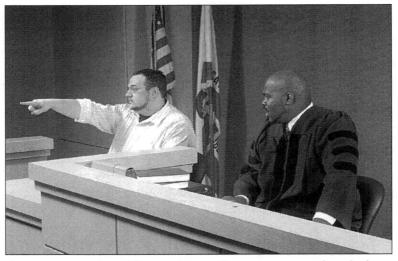

Any time you use physical force against another person, you run the risk of having a civil suit filed against you. Always be certain you actions are legally warranted in the eyes of the law.

With that being said, there are two primary factors that determine the lethality of a cane strike. They are:

- **The anatomical target that you select.**
- **The amount of force you deliver to the intended target.**

The following chart will give you an idea of which anatomical targets are considered to be lethal.

Lethal Targets	Nonlethal Targets
Eyes	Nose
Temple	Chin
Throat	Collarbone
Back of Neck	Ribs
Spine	Solar Plexus
	Groin
	Thighs/Knees
	Shins
	Elbows
	Hands

Cane Target Orientation

The most effective way for developing target orientation is to practice cane strikes on the body opponent bag or BOB.

The body opponent bag is a self-standing lifelike punching bag designed to withstand tremendous punishment by allowing you to attack it with a wide variety of offensive techniques.

Because of its lifelike features, the body opponent bag is ideal for developing accuracy with your strikes. The following photos will show you the various targets on the bag.

Front View Targets

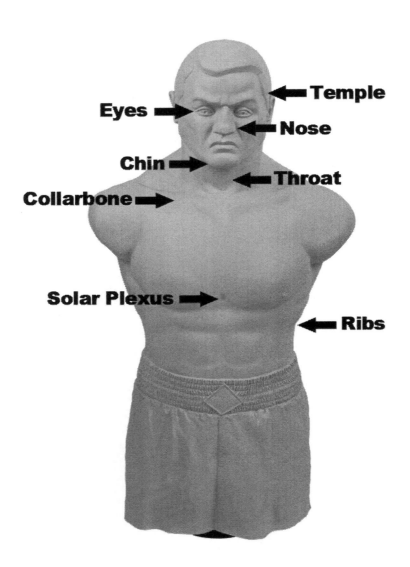

Side View Targets

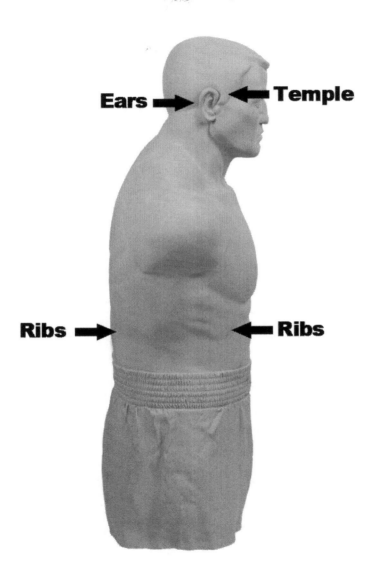

Rear View Targets

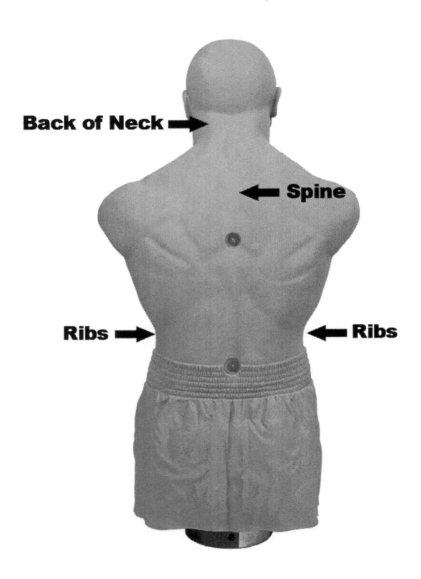

Target Recognition

The next component of target awareness is called target recognition. Target Recognition is the ability to immediately recognize specific targets during the actual confrontation, including both the precontact and contact stages of self-defense.

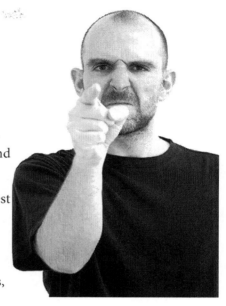

As I discussed earlier, the best targets for the cane are sensitive bony and soft tissue parts of the body like the eyes, temple, nose, chin, back of neck, throat, hands, etc.

Target recognition requires that you keep your calm during the duress of a combat situation and maintain a complete visual picture of your adversary.

One of the biggest mistakes that you can make during a fight is to gaze or stare into your opponent's eyes. Looking steadily into the assailant's eyes will significantly restricts your ability to recognize target opportunities during a fight.

One of the best ways to develop target recognition is to regularly participate in role-playing scenarios that replicate the stress of a real-world self-defense situations. A good reality based self-defense instructor can help you with this.

Target Selection

The third component of target awareness is target selection. When using a walking stick for personal defense, never strike the opponent with reckless abandon. All of your blows must be smart and calculated. Target selection is the cognitive process of selecting the appropriate anatomical target to strike in combat.

Selecting the appropriate target is predicated on three important factors:

1. **Proximity of Opponent** - how far is the opponent from your cane?

2. **Positioning of Opponent** - exactly where is the opponent positioned and at what angle and height from your cane?

3. **Use of Force** - the amount of force that is legally warranted for this particular self-defense situation. Remember, not every self-defense situation will warrant using deadly force. This means that you are not permitted or justified to strike deadly force targets. Deadly force targets include the eyes, temple, throat, back of neck, and the spinal column.

Target Impaction

Target Impaction is the physical process of striking the selected target with your weapon. Target impaction requires that each and every blow be delivered with maximum speed and power and minimal telegraphing. Proper attribute development will ensure successful target impaction during a confrontation.

Again, practicing regularly on the body opponent bag will help you develop the necessary speed and power required for effective cane striking technique.

Target Exploitation

Finally, once you have acquired target impaction, you can implement target exploitation. Target exploitation is a combative attribute that allows you to strategically exploit your assailant's reaction dynamics during the altercation.

For example, let's say you successfully strike your opponent in the solar plexus with your cane and the impact from your attack causes the adversary to bend forward in pain. The opponent's physical action of bending over is called a "reaction dynamic."

Target exploitation allows you to take advantage of the opponent's reaction dynamic by following up with another logical strike. In this case, a knee strike to the face would be an excellent follow up technique.

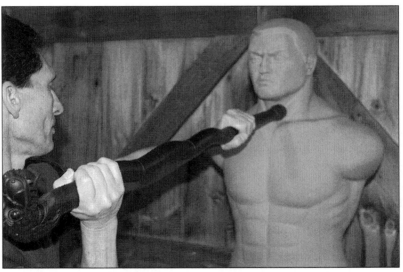

Successful target impaction requires you to practice your cane strikes on a con-sistent basis. Remember, repetition is the mother of skill!

Other Cane Fighting Attributes

While target awareness is a vital attribute for cane fighting, there are others that are just as important and certainly worth mentioning.

Speed

In both armed and unarmed fighting you have to be fast- real fast! Your offensive and defensive techniques must move like a flash of lightening.

Actually, speed is a chief fighting attribute necessary for reality based self-defense. What most people don't realize is, fighting speed is something that you can easily improve. There are specific drills and exercises or speed training that can dramatically boost the quickness of your cane techniques as well as other fighting moves.

Combat speed is much like a steel chain made up of several separate links that are related to one another. Each link in the combat speed chain represents a particular component or unique attribute of quickness that must be practiced to maximize the overall acceleration of your martial arts skills and abilities.

One of the most effective methods of enhancing the physical speed of your cane fighting techniques is to avoid tensing your body and simply relaxing your muscles prior to executing your movement.

Another way of developing blistering speed is to practice a particular cane strike thousands of times until the motor movement is sharpened and crystallized. I know this might sound boring, but I can assure you it produces great results.

Striking Power

When it come to real world self-defense, you must be capable of striking your opponent with knock-out force. To put it more bluntly, you've got to knock him on his ass!

Striking power refers to the amount of force you can generate when striking with your stick. Contrary to popular belief, striking power is not simply predicated on size, strength or body weight. There are other significant factors like power generator mastery, follow-through, and tool velocity that also play a critical role.

For example, one crucial factor of striking power is learning to develop proper technique or "body mechanics" and it can be accomplished through proper training.

Also, learning to use your three anatomical power generators will allow you to generate tremendous force when striking the adversary.

Essentially, power generators are specific points on your body which help generate impact power They are:

- **Feet**

- **Hips**

- **Shoulders**

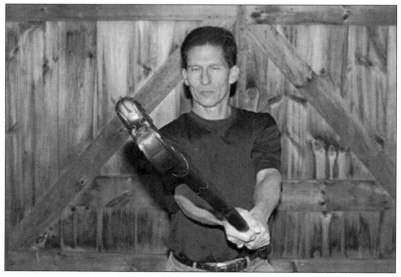

Putting your entire body behind your strike will maximize the impact power of your cane strike.

Cane Fighting

Maximally torquing your body into your cane strikes will significantly increase both the force and penetration of the blow.

Balance

Balance is the ability to maintain equilibrium while attacking and defending. You can maintain your balance in combat by controlling your center of gravity, mastering body mechanics and maintaining proper skeletal alignment.

To develop a better sense of balance, perform your cane strikes slowly in front of a mirror so you become acquainted with the different weight distributions, body positions, and mechanics of each particular technique.

Also, remember that balance is often lost due to weak body mechanics, poor kinesthetic perception, unnecessary weight shifting, excessive follow-through and improper skeletal alignment.

Non-Telegraphic Movement

It's critical not to telegraph or forewarn your opponent of your intentions to strike. Telegraphing means inadvertently making your offensive intentions known to your adversary.

In street self-defense, you must posses clean body mechanics that don't inform your adversary of your combative agenda. Basically, all of your movements have be non-telegraphic.

There are many forms of telegraphing which need to be purged from your cane fighting arsenal. Here are a few examples:

- Staring at your selected target.
- Chambering your arm back before striking.
- Tensing any part of your body prior to striking.
- Grinning or opening your mouth.

- Widening your eyes or raising your eyebrows.
- Taking a sudden, deep breath.

Relaxation

Your body must be relaxed (but ready) during a threatening situation. You must also be free from muscular tension and the psychological pressure of combat. There are several effective ways to reduce nervous tension and enhance physical relaxation during a fight.

- **Preparation** - be prepared to handle the myriad of personal defense situations.

- **Proper breathing** - control and pace your breathing during the threatening encounter.

- **Fight-or-flight response** - learn to accept and control your fight-or-flight response during the altercation.

- **Proper attitude** - always maintain a positive attitude during a threatening situation.

- **Kinesthetic perception** - kinesthetic perception is important because it allows you to effectively regulate or monitor the muscular tension in your body when fighting.

Cane Fighting

Chapter Five
Cane Striking Techniques

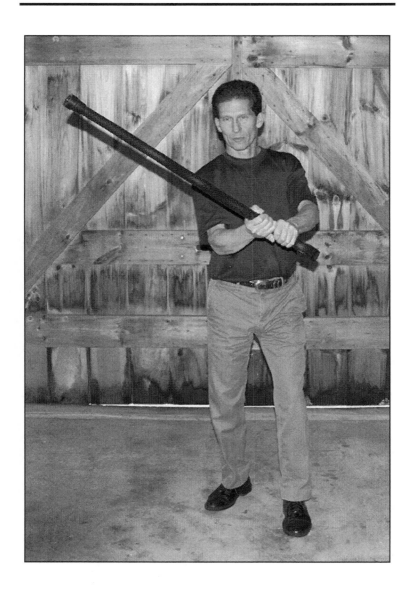

It's Time For a Reality Check

Chapter 1 discussed some of the inherent dangers of impractical cane fighting techniques, and it bears repeating. Do not attempt trapping, hooking, or pinning techniques with your cane. They are just too complicated, unreliable and inefficient to use against a non-compliant adversary who is fueled by either drugs, rage or adrenaline.

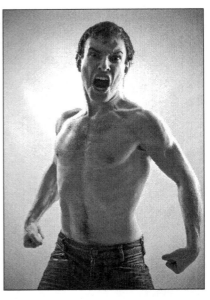

Remember, on the streets, there is no bushido, the honorable code of the ancient warrior. There are no rules of combat etiquette. Real life situations of violence are bloody, unpredictable, and extremely dangerous.

The tricky or flashy cane fighting moves that might look functional in movies or television will get you severely injured or possibly killed when defending against a powerful adversary who is hell-bent on destroying you.

Reality based cane fighting techniques must be efficient, effective and provide the least amount of danger are risk for the practitioner. Each and every physical movement must be strictly devoted to defending the sanctity of your space and body and perhaps ultimately your life.

As I said before, *the true combat utility of any tactical cane is to stop your attacker dead in his tracks through the application of blunt force trauma to specific vulnerable targets.* It's that plain and simple!

You Must Strike with Two Hands

As I stated in Chapter 2, you can safely use a one hand grip under very limited circumstances (i.e., fist loading or delivering a preemptive strike). However, the vast majority of your cane strikes should be performed with both of your hands held firmly on the stick. This essential rule is necessary for two important reasons:

1. **Knockout Power**

2. **Weapon Retention**

Despite what others might say, you cannot generate sufficient neutralizing impact power with a one-handed cane strike. Even under the best of conditions, it won't stop a powerful and determined adversary. This fact is especially true for seniors and other individuals who don't possess the size and strength to generate neutralizing power with one hand.

Weapon retention is another concern. If you strike your attacker with a one hand grip, you run the risk of your assailant grabbing your weapon with two hands and pulling it away from you.

To further illustrate my point, here are just a few self-defense scenarios that would render a one-handed cane strike useless:

- Defending against an attacker who is high on psychoactive drugs.

- Defending against a psychotic or mentally ill person.

- Defending against an attacker who "goes postal."

- Defending against trained fighters (boxer, mixed martial artists, etc.) who possess a high level of pain tolerance.

- Defending against adrenaline fueled attackers.

- Defending against an attacker who is wearing protective clothing like a thick leather jacket or heavy winter coat.

The Nine Cane Striking Angles

To efficiently administer blunt force trauma with a cane or walking stick, you must have a foundational understanding of the nine striking angles. Interestingly enough, these are the very same striking angles that are used in both single and double stick combat.

Let's take a closer look at each angle of attack. We will start with angle 1.

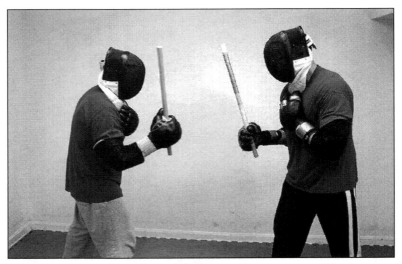

The nine striking angles used in stick fighting are the same ones used for the tactical cane. Pictured here, two students square off during a stick fight.

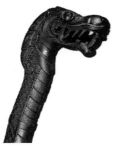

Regular stick fighting training with dramatically improve both your offensive and defensive reaction time. This is because the rattan stick travels up to five times faster than the hands. Don't neglect this essential form of self-defense training!

Angle 1

Angle One is a diagonal forehand strike traveling from right to left. Impact can be made with the handle, knob, or shaft of your cane. Anatomical targets include your assailant's temple, clavicle, back of neck, spine, elbow, ribs, thigh, knee joint, shins, and hands.

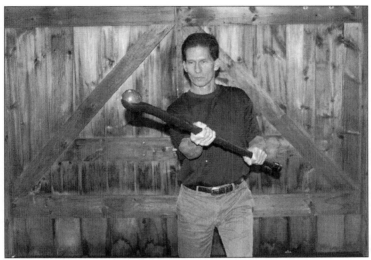

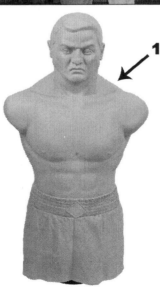

Angle 2

Angle Two is a diagonal backhand strike traveling from left to right. Impact can be made with the handle, knob, or shaft of your cane. Anatomical targets include your assailant's temple, clavicle, back of neck, spine, elbow, ribs, thigh, knee joint, shins, and hands.

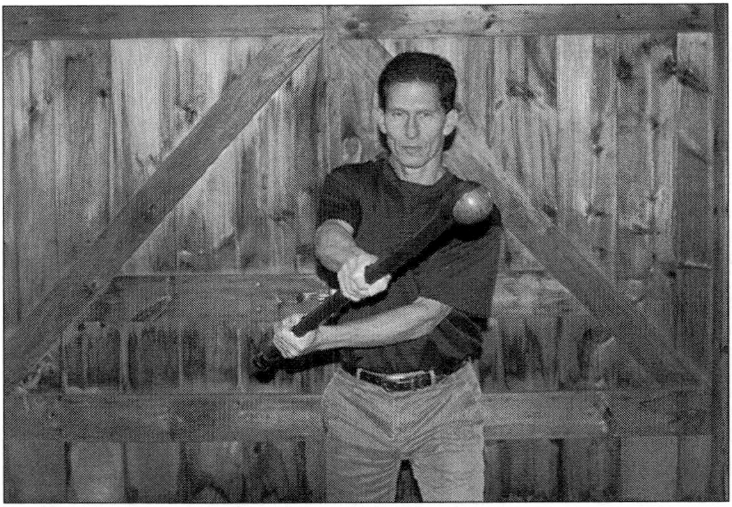

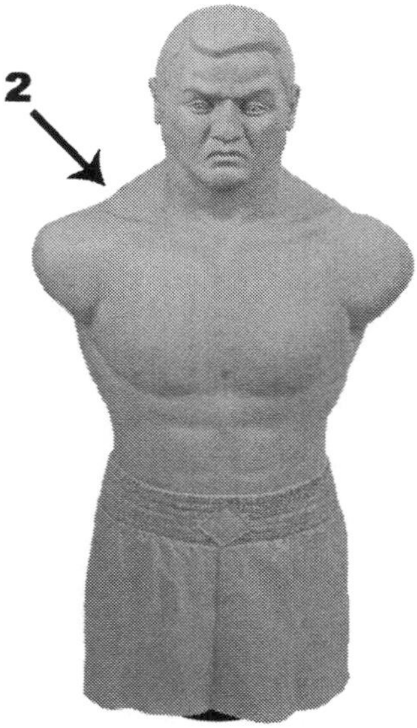

Angle 3

Angle Three is a horizontal forehand strike traveling from right to left. Impact can be made with the handle, knob, or shaft of your cane. Anatomical targets include your assailant's temple, back of neck, spine, elbow, ribs, thigh, shins, knee joint, and hands.

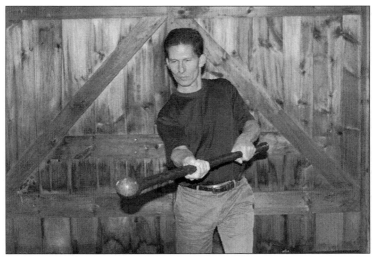

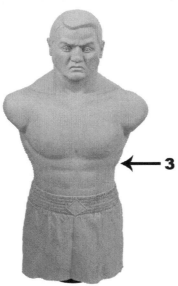

Angle 4

Angle Four is a horizontal backhand strike traveling from left to right. Impact is made with either the handle, knob, or shaft of your cane. Anatomical targets include your assailant's temple, back of neck, spine, elbow, ribs, thigh, shins, knee joint, and hands.

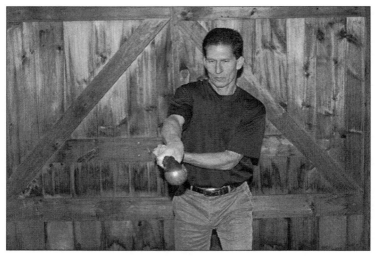

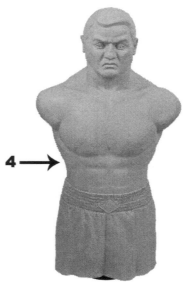

Angle 5

Angle Five is an upward diagonal forehand moving from right to left. Impact is made with either the handle, knob, or shaft of your cane. Anatomical targets include your assailant's temple, chin, elbow, ribs, thigh, shins, knee joint, and hands.

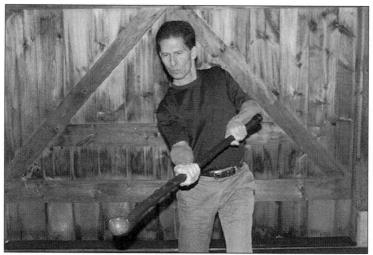

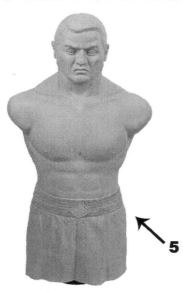

Angle 6

Angle Six is an upward diagonal backhand strike moving from left to right. Impact is made with either the handle, knob, or shaft of your cane. Anatomical targets include your assailant's temple, chin, elbow, ribs, thigh, shins, knee joint, and hands.

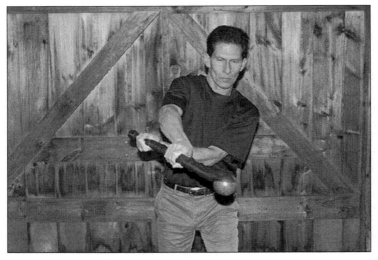

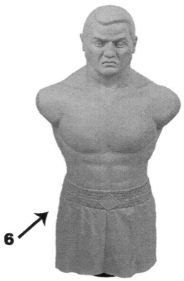

Angle 7

Angle Seven is a linear thrust delivered anywhere on the assailant's centerline. Impact is made with tip of your cane. Anatomical targets include your assailant's face, eyes, throat, solar plexus, spine, back of neck, and groin.

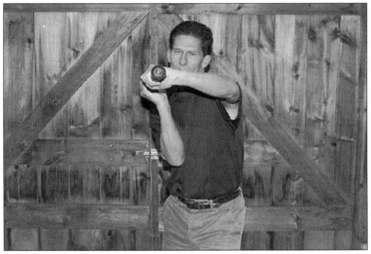

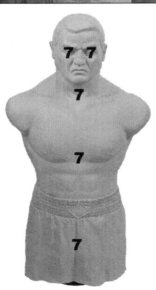

Angle 8

Angle Eight is a downward vertical strike. Impact is made with either the handle, knob, shaft, or tip of your cane. Anatomical targets include your assailant's head, clavicle, back of neck, spine, elbow, ribs, thigh, knee joint, and hands.

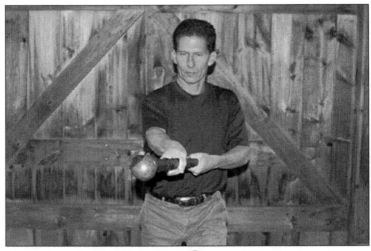

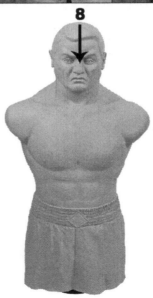

Angle 9

Angle Nine is an upward vertical strike. Impact is made with either the handle, knob, or shaft of your cane. Anatomical targets include your assailant's chin, elbow, ribs, groin, thigh, knee joint, and hands.

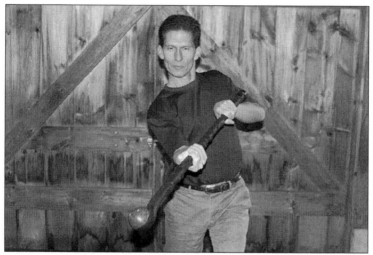

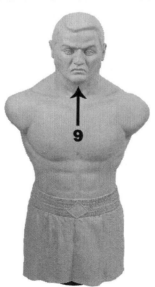

The Nine Cane Striking Angles

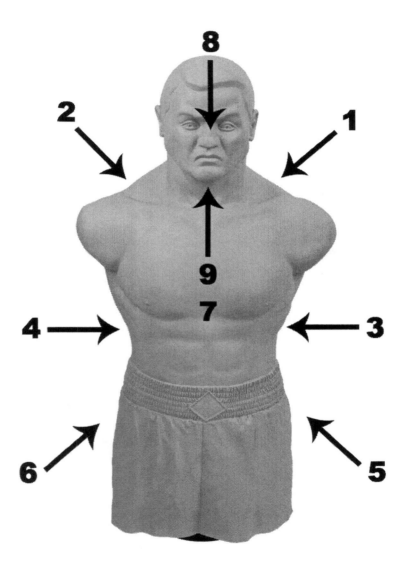

The Importance of Combining Striking Angles

It most self-defense situations it will take more than just a single strike to stop your attacker. In fact, you will almost always have to initiate a strategic compound attack.

A compound attack is what immediately follows your initial cane strike, and it's defined as the logical sequence of two or more strikes strategically thrown in succession. The objective is to take the fight out of the assailant and the assailant out of the fight by destroying his defenses with a burst of full-force strikes.

Based on speed, power, target selection, and target exploitation, the compound attack also requires calculation, precision, and clarity. To maximize your compound attack, you must have a thorough knowledge and awareness of the anatomical targets presented by your adversary. Remember, unless your assailant is in full body armor, there are always targets. It is simply a question of your selecting them and attacking quickly with the appropriate cane strikes.

Probable Reaction Dynamics (PRD)

In my book, *Maximum Damage: Hidden Secrets Behind Brutal Fighting Combinations*, I define probable reaction dynamics as the opponent's anticipated or predicted movements or actions that occur in both armed and unarmed combat. Probable reaction dynamics will always be the result or residual of your initial action, i.e., cane strike, punch, kick, etc.

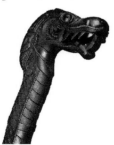

Probable reaction dynamics will always be the result or residual of your initial action. This action can be in the form of a verbal statement, physical technique, or simple gesture directed at your opponent.

Cane Fighting

The most basic example of probable reaction dynamics can be illustrated by the following scenario. Let's say, you forcefully drive the tip of your cane into his groin. When your cane comes in contact with its target, your opponent will exhibit one of several *possible* physical or psychological reactions to your strike. These responses might include:

- The opponent's head and body violently drop forward.
- The opponent grabs or covers his groin region.
- The opponent struggles for breath.
- The opponent momentarily freezes.
- The opponent goes into shock.

Knowledge of your assailant's probable reaction dynamics is vital in all forms of combat, including cane fighting. In fact, you must be mindful of the possible reaction dynamics to every strike, and technique in your arsenal. This is exactly what I refer to as *"reaction dynamic awareness"* and I can assure you this is not such an easy task. However, with regular training, it can be developed.

Just remember, understanding and ultimately mastering reaction dynamic awareness will give you a tremendous advantage in a fight by maximizing the effectiveness, efficiency and safety of your compound attack.

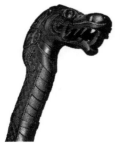

Breathing is one of the most important and often neglected aspects of self-defense. Proper breathing promotes muscular relaxation and increases the speed and efficiency of your compound attack. The rate at which you breathe will also determine how quickly your body can recover from a violent encounter.

Flow Like Water!

When you proceed with the compound attack, always maintain the offensive flow. The offensive flow is a progression of continuous offensive movements designed to neutralize or, in some cases, terminate your adversary. The key is to have each cane strike flow smoothly and efficiently from one to the next without causing you to lose ground. Subjecting your adversary to an offensive flow is especially effective because it taxes his nervous system, thereby dramatically lengthening his defensive reaction time.

In a real-life emergency situation it's critical that you always keep the offensive pressure on until your opponent is completely neutralized. Always remember that letting your offensive flow stagnate, even for a second, will open you up to numerous dangers and risks.

Proper breathing is another substantial element of the compound attack, and there is one simple rule that should be followed: exhale during the execution phase of your cane strike and inhale during its retraction phase. Above all, never hold your breath when delivering several consecutive blows. Doing so could lead to dizziness and fainting, among other complications.

You Don't Have Much Time

Your body can only sustain delivering a compound attack for so long. Initially, your brain will quickly release adrenaline into your blood stream, which will fuel your fighting and enhance your strength and power. This lethal boost of energy is known as an adrenaline dump. However, your ability to exert and maintain this maximum effort will last no more than 30 to 60 seconds if you are in above-average shape. If the fight continues after that, your strength and speed may drop by as much as 50 percent below normal. When all is said and done, you don't have much time in a fight, so the battle needs to be won fast before your energy runs out!

Don't Forget To Relocate!

Subsequent to your compound attack, immediately move to a new location by flanking your adversary. This tactic is known as relocating. Based on the principles of strategy, movement, and surprise, relocating dramatically enhances your safety by making it difficult for your adversary to identify your position after you have attacked him. Remember, if your opponent doesn't know exactly where you are, he won't be able to effectively counterattack.

Actuate Recovery Breathing

Implementing an explosive compound attack will often leave you winded. Because of the volatile nature of street combat, even highly conditioned fighters will show signs of oxygen debt. Hence it's important to employ recovery breathing, the active process of quickly restoring your breathing to its normal state. It requires taking long, deep breaths in a controlled rhythm while avoiding rapid, short gasping. Wind sprints are great for improving your recovery breathing. Consider adding them to your regular training program.

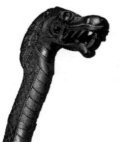

Since most people often associate a cane with a disability, you'll have the element of surprise when you to use it during a self-defense situation.

Cane Combination Examples
Combination One: Angle 1- Angle 2 - Angle 7

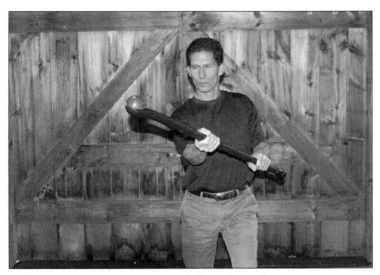

Step 1: Begin with the angle 1 strike.

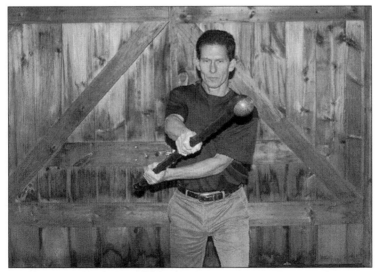

Step 2: Next, the angle 2 strike.

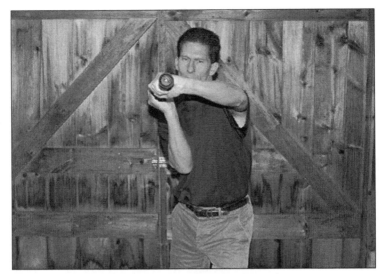

Step 3: Follow up with the angle 7 strike.

Combination Two: Angle 1- Angle 2 - Angle 3 - Angle 4

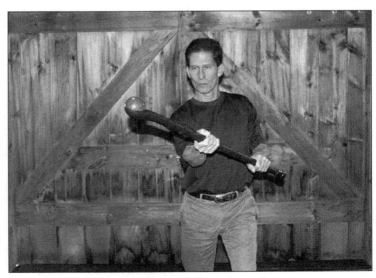

Step 1: Begin with the angle 1 strike.

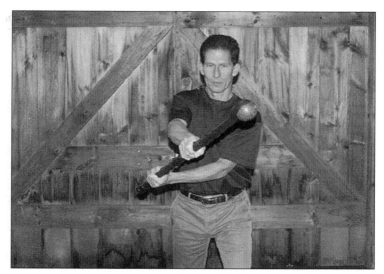

Step 2: Next, the angle 2 strike.

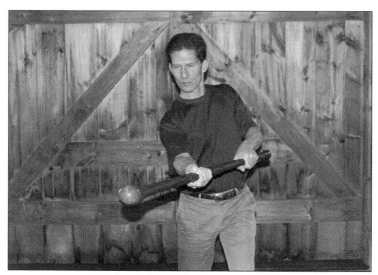

Step 3: Follow up with angle 3.

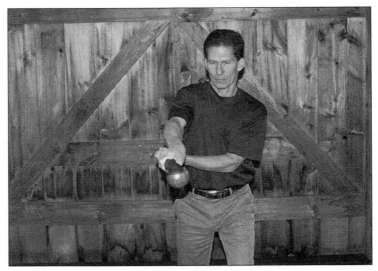

Step 4: Finish with the angle 4 strike.

Combination Three: Angle 7- Angle 8 - Angle 9

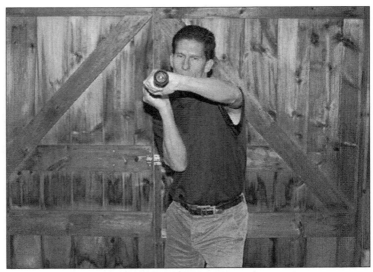

Step 1: Begin with the angle 7 strike.

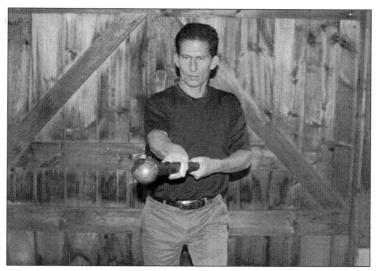

Step 2: Next, attack with the angle 8 strike.

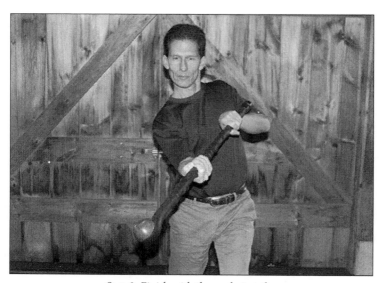

Step 3: Finish with the angle 9 strike.

Combination Four: Angle 3- Angle 4 - Angle 3 - Angle 4

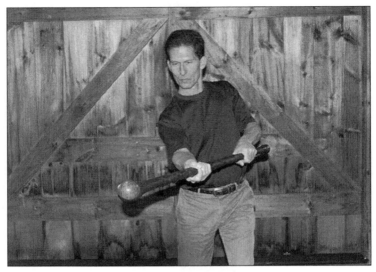

Step 1: Begin with angle 3.

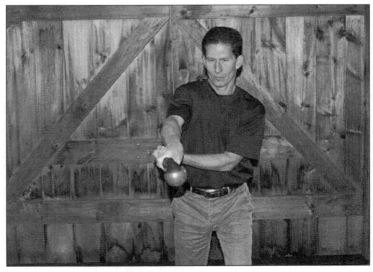

Step 2: Next, the angle 4 strike.

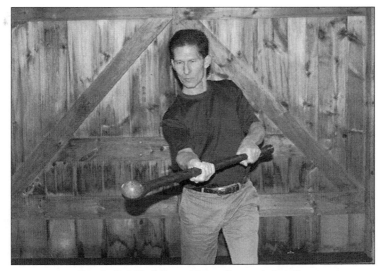

Step 3: Quickly follow with another angle 3 strike.

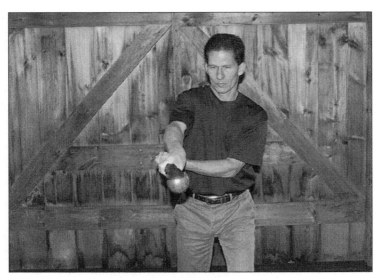

Step 4: Finish with angle 4.

Combination Five: Angle 1- Angle 2 - Angle 5 - Angle 6

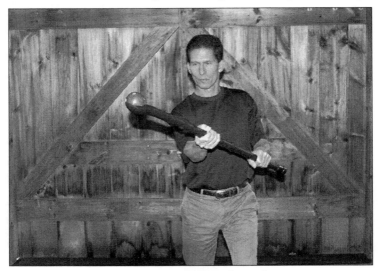

Step 1: Begin with the angle 1 strike.

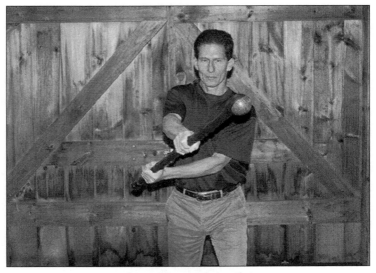

Step 2: Next, angle 2 strike.

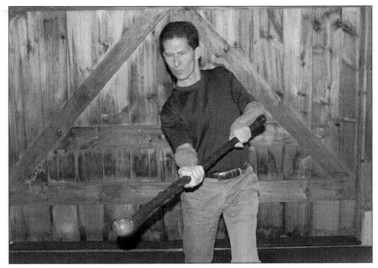

Step 3: Follow up with angle 5.

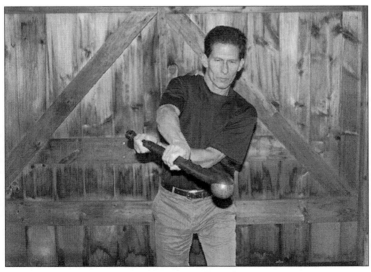

Step 4: Finish with angle 6.

Combination Six: Angle 8- Angle 9 - Angle 8 - Angle 9

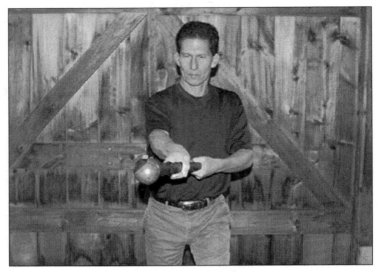

Step 1: Start with angle 8.

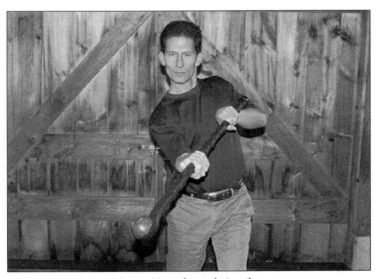

Step 3: Next, the angle 9 strike.

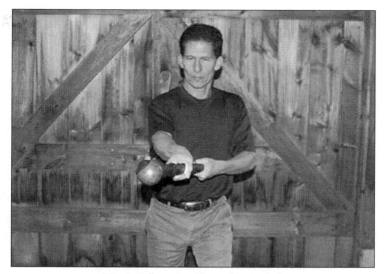

Step 3: Follow up with another angle 8.

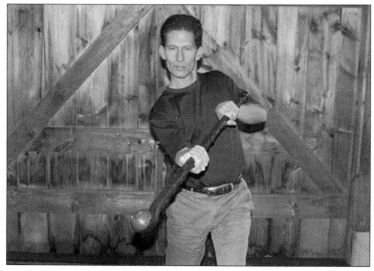

Step 4: Finish with the angle 9 strike.

Combination Seven: Angle 7- Angle 7 - Angle 9 - Angle 4

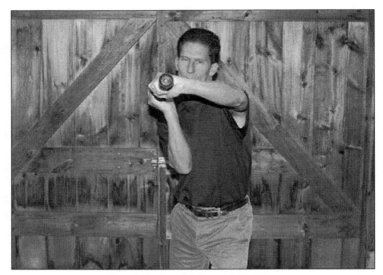

Step 1: Begin with the angle 7 strike.

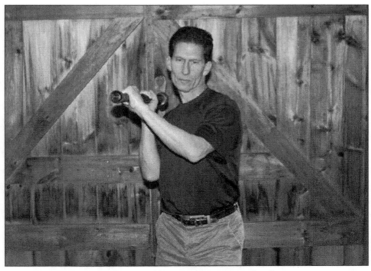

Step 2: Quickly retract your arms back.

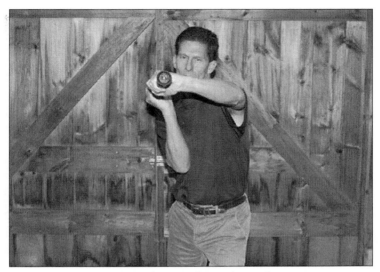

Step 3: Deliver another angle 7 strike.

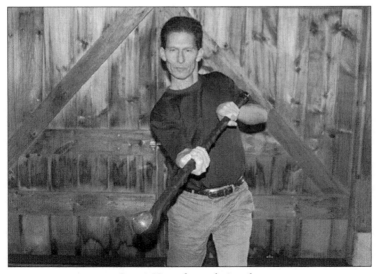

Step 4: Next, the angle 9 strike.

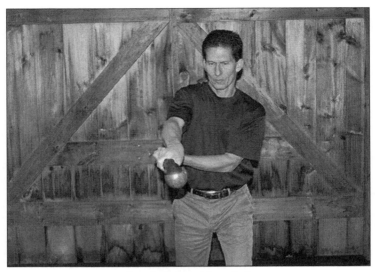

Step 5: Finish with angle 4.

Combination Eight: Angle 5- Angle 6 - Angle 3 - Angle 4 - Angle 9

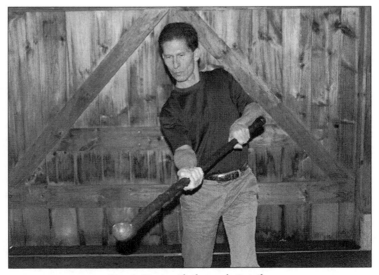

Step 1: Start with the angle 5 strike.

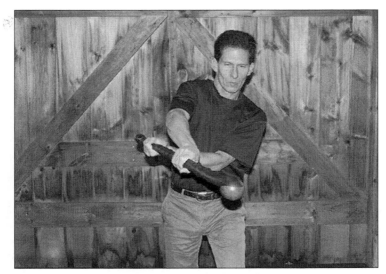

Step 2: Next, the angle 6 strike.

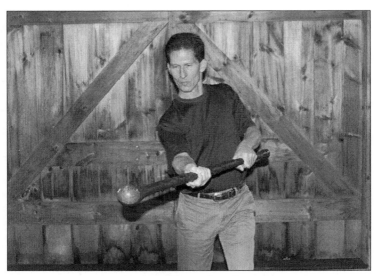

Step 3: Follow with angle 3.

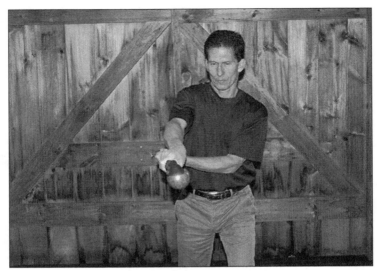

Step 4: Deliver the angle 4 strike.

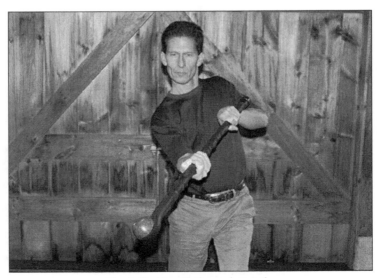

Step 5: Finish with the angle 9 strike.

Combination Nine: Angle 1- Angle 6 - Angle 5 - Angle 2 - Angle 7

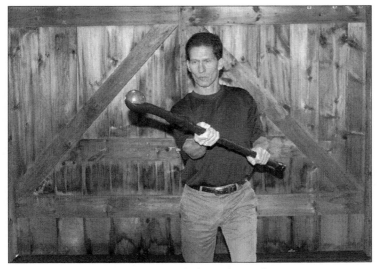

Step 1: Begin with the angle 1 strike.

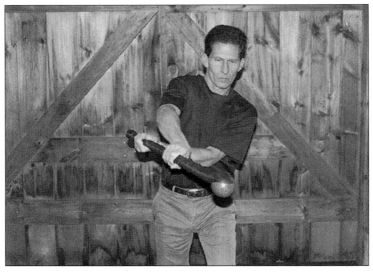

Step 2: Next, the angle 6 strike.

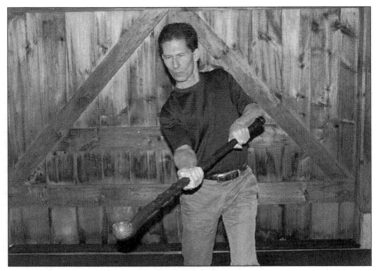

Step 3: Follow with the angle 5 strike.

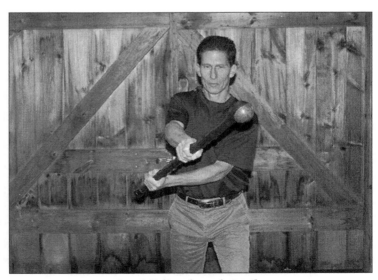

Step 4: Deliver the angle 2 strike.

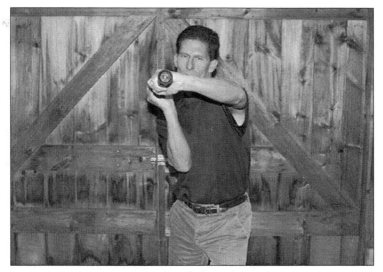

Step 5: Finish with the angle 7 strike.

Combination Ten: Angles 1 through 9

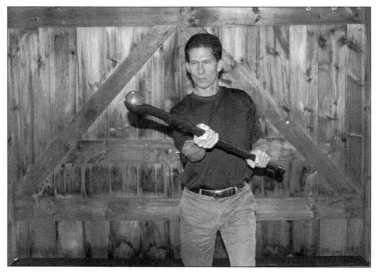

Step 1: Begin with the angle 1 strike.

115

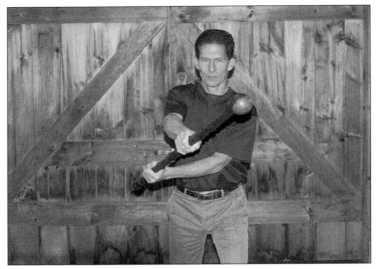

Step 2: Next, the angle 2 strike.

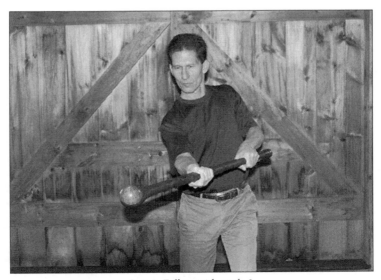

Step 3: Follow with angle 3.

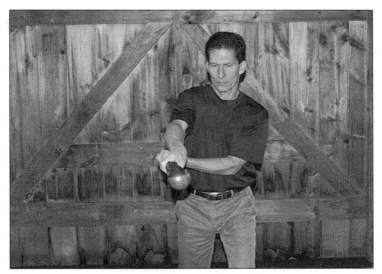

Step 4: Deliver the angle 4 strike.

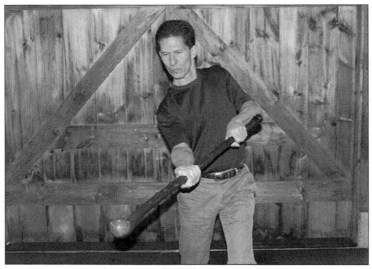

Step 5: Follow up with the angle 5 strike.

117

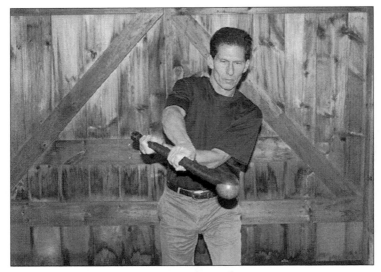

Step 6: Angle 6 strike.

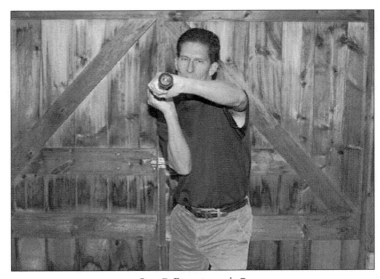

Step 7: Execute angle 7.

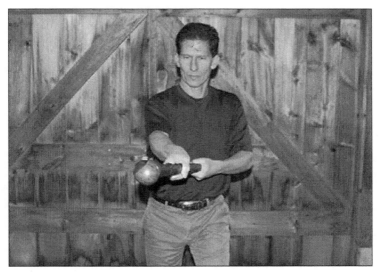

Step 8: Follow up with angle 8.

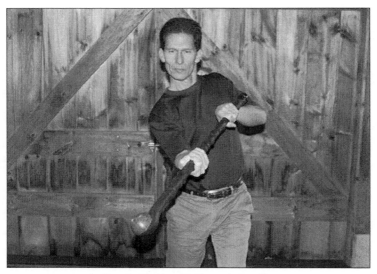

Step 9: Finish with the angle 9 strike.

Cane Fighting

Create Your Own Cane Fighting Combinations

To get you into the process of developing your own striking combinations, I have provided a section for you to write them down. Remember, be creative!

1.

2.

3.

4.

5.

6.

7.

8.

9.

10.

11.

12.

13.

14.

15.

16.

17.

18.

19.

20.

21.

22.

23.

24.

25.

26.

27.

28.

29.

30.

31.

32.

33.

34.

35.

36.

37.

38.

39.

40.

Be Careful With Power Swings

A word of caution when attempting a full-power swing at your opponent. Since a power swing requires your cane to travels 180 degrees across your body, it creates momentary areas of vulnerability that can be exploited by a skilled adversary.

To better understand the inherent vulnerability of a power swing, we can divide the movement into three phases. They are:

1. **Initiation phase** - the starting point of your swing.

2. **Mid phase** - the contact point of your swing, where your cane impacts the target.

3. **Completion phase** - the end point of your swing.

Just be aware that your assailant can move in and *choke* your swing during either the initiation or completion phases of your strike.

The Three Phases of a Power Swing

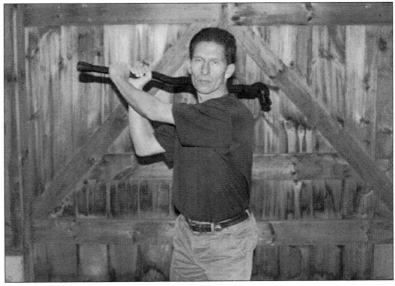

Step 1: The initiation phase of your swing.

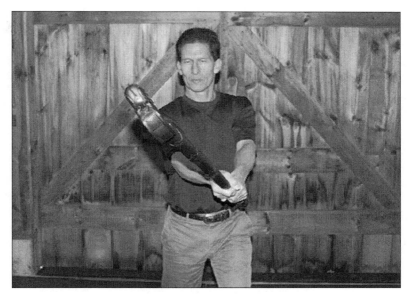

Step 2: The mid-phase of your swing.

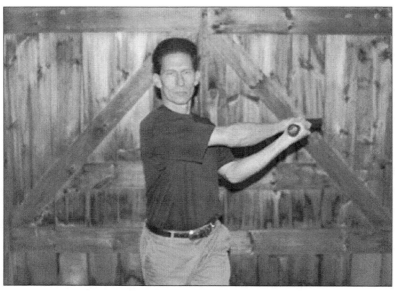

Step 3: The completion phase of your swing.

Preventing a Power Swing Choke

The best way to prevent your power swing from being choked is to avoid telegraphing your attack. Telegraphing means inadvertently making your intentions known to your assailant. There are many subtle forms of telegraphing that must be avoided when using your cane during a high-risk self-defense situation. Here are just a few:

1. Demonstratively cocking your arms back prior to striking with your cane.

2. Tensing your neck, shoulders, or arms prior to striking.

3. Widening your eyes or raising your eyebrows.

4. Shifting your shoulders.

5. Grinning or opening your mouth.

6. Taking a sudden, deep breath.

One of the most effective ways to prevent telegraphing movement is to maintain a poker face prior to executing your offensive movements. Actually you should avoid all facial expressions when faced with a threatening adversary. You can also study your cane fighting techniques and movements in front of a full-length mirror or have a training partner video your movements. These training procedures will assist you in identifying and ultimately eliminating telegraphic movement from your cane fighting arsenal.

Essential Cane Striking Strategies

Here are some valuable tips that will help improve your cane striking techniques.

Watch Your Centerline

When engaged in cane fighting, avoid exposing your centerline unnecessarily. Not only does this expose your vital targets to your adversary, it also diminishes your balance and inhibits efficient footwork. During any emergency self-defense situation, try to maintain a 45-degree stance in relation to your adversary.

Don't Hold Your Cane Too Tightly

You should apply a moderate amount of pressure when gripping your cane. Grasping it too tightly can be problematic for the following reasons:

1. It will tire your hands and cause unnecessary cramping.

2. It may telegraph your striking movements.

3. It will significantly reduce the speed of your strikes.

4. It will reduce the power of your strikes.

5. It will throw off your offensive and defensive timing.

Defend From Different Positions

There are nine general positions in which you can fight your adversary with your cane. They include the following:

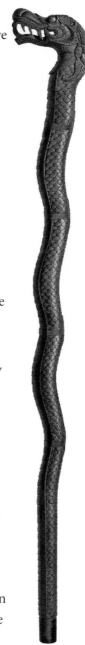

Cane Fighting

1. Both you and your assailant are prone.

2. You are kneeling and your assailant is prone.

3. Your assailant is kneeling and you are prone.

4. Both you and your assailant are kneeling.

5. You are standing and your assailant is prone.

6. Your assailant is standing and you are prone.

7. You are standing and your assailant is kneeling.

8. Your assailant is standing and you are kneeling.

9. Both you and your assailant are standing.

Follow Through With Your Cane Strike

When striking your adversary, always follow-through with your blow. The follow-through strike is the most effective strike for stick combat because it creates the necessary amount of force to incapacitate your adversary.

Keep Your Elbow Slightly Bent When Swinging

When delivering a blow with your walking stick, keep your elbow slightly bent. This rule of thumb is important for the following reasons:

1. It prevents hyperextension of your elbows.

2. It enhances the speed of your strike.

3. It enhances the power of your blow.

4. It reduces telegraphing your strike.

5. It helps control the arc of your swing.

6. It minimizes your target exposure.

Avoid Overextending Your Swing

Avoid overextending the arc of your swing for some of the following reasons.

1. It's easier for your assailant to defend against an long arc swing.

2. It slows down the speed of your blow.

3. You can possibly hyperextend your elbow when impact is made with your target.

4. It lacks sufficient neutralizing power.

5. It promotes telegraphic movement.

6. Your adversary can easily evade your strike.

7. It maximizes target exposure to your adversary.

Cane Retention is a Vital Skill

When engaged in a personal defense situation, avoid dropping or losing control of your weapon. Here are some important reasons why:

1. If your assailant is already armed with a weapon he will now have a huge tactical advantage.

2. If your assailant is unarmed, he can pick up your cane and use it against you.

3. Spectators can attack you with it.

4. You can possibly trip over it, lose your balance and fall.

Keep Your Cane Moving

Once the actual fight begins, try to keep both you and your defensive cane moving. This is important for the following reasons:

1. It prevents inertia from setting in and slowing you down.

2. Movement enhances the overall velocity of your cane strikes.

3. It helps minimizes telegraphing prior to striking.

4. It enhances your defensive reaction time.

5. It minimizes your hand and digit exposure in the event your attacker wants to attack your hands.

6. It significantly enhances your offensive flow during the course of your compound attack.

7. It helps your assailant misjudge your weapon's range.

Improving Your Cane Fighting Speed

There are several ways you can increase the speed of your cane strikes. Here are just a few:

1. Once contact is made with the target, don't allow your strike to completely *settle* in the selected target.

2. When attacking, learn to step into the direction of your blow.

3. Repetition is the mother of skill. Practice various angles of attack thousands of times to sharpen and crystallize the movement.

4. Regularly visualize your cane strikes being delivered at blistering speed.

5. Avoid unnecessarily tensing your body and relax your muscles prior to the execution of your stick strike.

6. Remember to breathe when fighting and exhale during the execution of your strike.

7. Learn to *act* rather than react during an emergency self-

defense situation.

8.   Become one with your weapon and realize it's just an extension of your body.

9.   Try to apply moderate grip pressure when swinging your cane and tighten your grip when impact is made with the target.

10. Speed is a fighting attribute that is developed over time. Learn to be patient and you will be happy with your progress.

Cane Chokes

While this chapter is primarily devoted to efficient striking techniques, there are two different cane chokes that you can apply when faced with a deadly force self-defense situation.

However, a word of caution about choking techniques! Prolonged lack of oxygen to the brain may cause permanent injury or death. Cane chokes can be lethal and should only be used in situations that legally warrant the use of deadly force.

The American Choke Hold

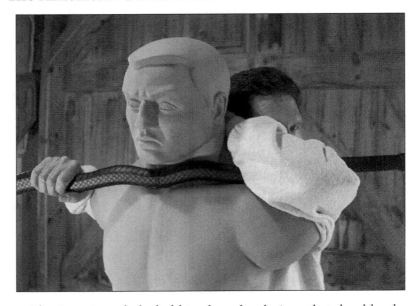

The American choke hold is a brutal technique that should only be used in life-or-death self-defense situations. To apply the choke, perform the following steps:

1. With your right hand, hold the cane in front of your assailant, parallel to the floor and against his throat.

2. Place your left arm (triceps area) over your adversary's left

shoulder while making certain that the shaft of your cane rests in the crook of your left elbow.

3. Place the palm of your left hand against the back of your assailant's neck.

4. In one fluid motion, apply pressure with your left hand against the back of your adversary's neck while simultaneously pulling your cane toward yourself with your right hand.

5. Keep the side of your head pressed against the back of your left hand throughout the execution of the movement.

The Ice Pick Choke Hold

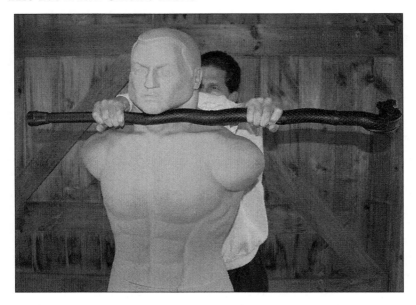

The ice-pick choke hold is another devastating cane fighting technique that can be applied with minimal effort. This choke can be lethal and should be used only in life-and-death self-defense situations when lethal force is warranted.

Cane Fighting

To apply the strangle, follow these important steps:

1. Standing behind your assailant with your cane in your right hand.

2. With a one hand grip, insert the lower portion of your cane around the front of your assailant's neck from your left side.

3. Make certain that the shaft of the cane rests against the front of your assailant's throat and is parallel to the floor.

4. Cross your left arm over your right forearm and grasp the cane on the right side of your assailant's neck.

5. While making certain that both of your hands are close to the assailant's neck, apply immediate pressure by pulling both of your hands backward.

Warning! The ice-pick choke can easily crush the assailant's windpipe, causing death. Always be certain you actions are legally justified in the eyes of the law.

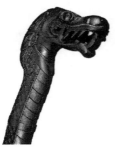

Notice how you don't need the hooked portion of a cane to perform these choking techniques.

Chapter Six
Defensive Techniques

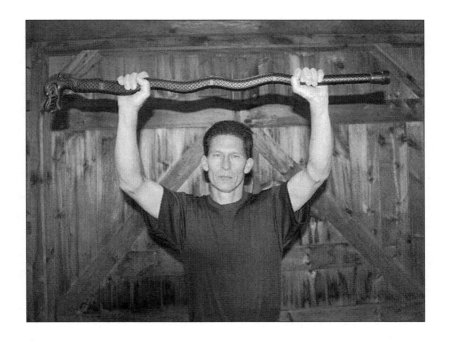

The Limitations of Defensive Cane Techniques

This book would be incomplete if I did not address defensive cane techniques. However, before discussing some of the skills and blocking maneuvers, it's important to inform you of one cold hard truth - the cane presents significant disadvantages during a self-defense situation.

As I stated throughout this book, the cane is a devastating offensive weapon capable of inflicting tremendous damage. However, as a defensive tool, it has limitations. Recognizing and understanding its weaknesses will go a long way in saving your life.

Committing Both Hands to the Cane

The greatest disadvantage of using a cane during a self-defense situation is that it requires two hands, basically tying both of them up during the fight. This is extremely dangerous for some of the following reasons:

The Postal Attack

One of the biggest concerns is facing a crazed assailant who *"goes postal"* and attacks you with an explosive and frenzied flurry of vicious blows. In most instances, your attacker will swing both of his arms wildly as he rushes or runs inexorably towards you.

There's no skill and no finesse involved with a postal attack.

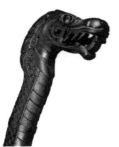

The slang term "going postal" was derived from a series of mass murder incidents that took in the United States Postal Service (USPS) from the mid 1980s to the mid 1990s.

THE "POSTAL ASSAULT"

- **Extremely fast**
- **Telegraphic form of attack**
- **Frenetic and awkward strikes**
- **Frequently delivered with both arms simultaneously**
- **Can override the defender's cognitive brain**
- **Assailant often screams when he attacks**
- **Assailant usually runs toward the defender**
- **Fueled by adrenaline, rage and fear**

Adrenaline, rage, and fear are the three primary ingredients that fuel his attack. However, psychoactive drugs like alcohol, amphetamines, cocaine, and PCP can also play an active role during a postal assault. Regardless, a person who goes postal will often look and act like an enraged madman hell-bent on destruction.

Going Postal is artless, but extremely dangerous for two reasons. One, the sudden outburst of violent energy often overrides the defender's cognitive brain, preventing him or her from applying the appropriate defensive technique at the proper moment. In most cases, the defender will freeze up, and this split-second of vulnerability is when he or she can get knocked out.

Two, the attack rhythm, angle, and trajectory of your opponent's assault are unpolished, uncoordinated and unpredictable. The punches are often frenetic and delivered at multiple awkward attack angles.

The bottom line is, defensive cane techniques won't stop someone who initiates a postal attack. It's just too fast and overwhelming for

Cane Fighting

the defender to effectively apply cane defense techniques. While you might be able to block one or two of the attacker's blows with your stick, the remainder of his postal attack will quickly steamroll over you.

What's more concerning is the fact that your average boxer, martial artist, or street thug can also overwhelm a cane-wielding defender with a simple, yet vicious, compound attack. Again, holding a cane or walking stick with both hands makes it virtually impossible to effectively block and parry the opponent's flurry of hand blows.

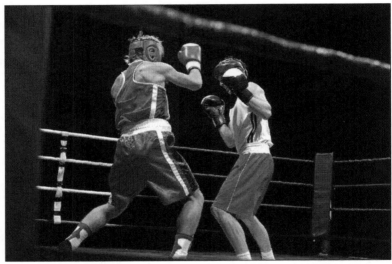

The postal attack is not your only threat. Even an amateur boxers has the firepower to overwhelm a cane fighter's defenses.

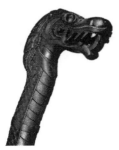

Going Postal is not just reserved for untrained people. There have been some instances where trained fighters, even well known martial arts grandmasters have "lost it" and gone postal in a street fight.

The Perfect Storm of Violence

The following photo sequence illustrates just how fast an attacker can close the distance gap during a postal attack. They often start out in a relatively calm state and quickly escalate to extreme rage within seconds.

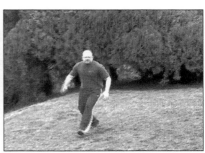

Step 1: Prior to his attack, the assailant nervously paces back and forth.

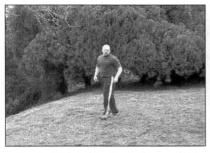

Step 2: He fixates on the defender and moves closer.

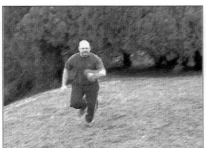

Step 3: Fueled by rage and adrenaline, the attacker explodes forward.

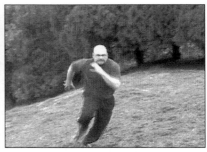

Step 4: He rushes at the defender like a freight train.

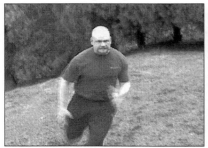

Step 5: The attacker raises his arms as he gets closer to his target.

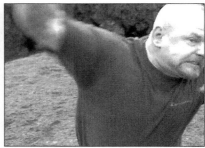

Step 6: As soon as he reaches striking distance, the barrage of blows begin.

Seeing The Postal Attack Before it Happens

You'll stand a much better chance of defending against a postal attack if you can see the impending danger before it happens. These few precious seconds might allow you to escape quickly from the dangerous situation or maybe attempt some smart de-escalation techniques.

Regardless, of which tactical option you choose, a properly trained self-defense technician must be aware of everything in their immediate surroundings, including the assailant's intentions to attack. He or she should possess the ability to recognize both verbal and nonverbal signs of impending aggression or assault. What follows is a list of both verbal and nonverbal indicators that violence is probable.

Verbal Indicators (Assault is imminent)

- Abnormal stuttering
- Rapid speech
- Incoherent speech
- Extreme sarcasm
- Threats
- Challenging statements
- Screaming and swearing

Nonverbal Indicators (Assault is possible)

- Increased breathing and pulse rate
- Excessive sweating
- Pulled shoulders
- Clenched teeth
- Direct and uninterrupted eye contact

- Acting as if he is ignoring you

- Drunken behavior

- Immediately changing from uncooperative to cooperative

Nonverbal Indicators (Assault is imminent)

- Clenched fists

- Quivering hands

- Cessation of all movements

- Reddened face (from blood surge)

- Protruding veins (from face, neck, or forearms)

- Extreme body tension

- Shoulder telegraph

- Target stare (looking at groin, jaw, etc.)

- Finger pointing

- Quick pacing

- Quick turning

- Fist threats with arm bent

- Hands on hips

- 1,000-yard stare (looking through you)

- Hand concealment

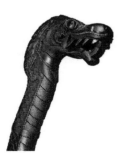

During the precontact stages of a self-defense altercation, it's more important to focus on what your opponent is doing, than what he is saying.

You Need Both Hands When Ground Fighting

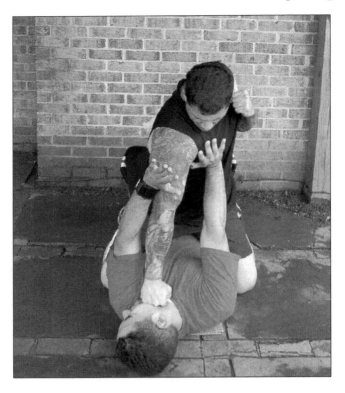

Regardless of how skilled you might be with your tactical cane, there's a good chance your adversary will force you to the ground during the fight. In fact, the majority of self-defense altercations (i.e., muggings, sexual assaults, barroom brawls, street fights, schoolyard fights, etc.) invariably end up on the ground.

A problem arises when you're armed with a cane and the adversary forces you to the ground. Aside from a couple choking techniques, the cane or walking stick is practically useless during a ground fight.

Surviving a ground fight requires that both of your hands are free to apply the many essential escapes, reversals, locks, holds, and chokes techniques. The cane or walking stick is simply too cumbersome for ground fighting. In almost every instance, you'll be forced to abandon your weapon to survive the ground fight.

Moreover, abandoning your cane during a ground fight creates another potential problem because there's always the possibility that belligerent spectators might decide to pick up your weapon and attack you with it.

You Need Both Hands to Defend Against a Knife

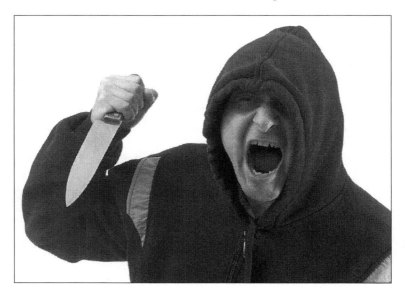

Let's be clear; the tactical cane is no match against a knife-wielding attacker. The notion that you can use your walking stick to smack a knife out of your attacker's hand is unrealistic. While this might happen in movies and television, it doesn't happen in the real world. Under the best of conditions, your cane might be able to keep your attacker away for a few precious seconds before he finally rushes you with a frenzied attack.

First, defending against a knife attack is extremely dangerous and should be avoided at all costs. In fact, if your situation presents the opportunity to safely escape, do it immediately!

Try to create as much distance as you can between you and the knife. Distance is critical because it enhances your defensive reaction time and allows you to control your options. Obviously, running away is an excellent way to put distance between you and the blade.

Nevertheless, if escaping is not an option, the number one rule when defending against a knife or edged weapon (i.e., a shard of glass, broken bottle, shank, etc.) is to always control the edged weapon first and then neutralize the assailant.

Again, holding a cane or walking stick occupies both of your hands, making it impossible to gain control of the assailant's knife. Remember, attempting to defend against a knife-wielding attacker while both of your hands are grasped firmly on your cane is foolish and will almost certainly get you killed.

In fact, the only effective method of controlling the assailant's knife hand is to use the V-grip. The V-grip is applied by grabbing the assailant's wrist (the one holding the knife) with **both of your hands** (make certain that the webs of your hands completely envelope your assailant's wrist). Once you have made contact, squeeze hard and hold on with all your might. When correctly applied, the V-grip will allow you to forcefully redirect the knife away from your body targets and effectively counter strike your adversary.

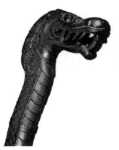

It's critical to make an accurate threat assessment when confronted by a knife-wielding assailant. Use split-second judgment to determine exactly what your adversary wants to accomplish. Some might not want to harm you if they can avoid it. Others may be dead-set on cutting you from limb to limb. If you have determined that your assailant plans to attack, you must resort to aggressive disarming tactics immediately.

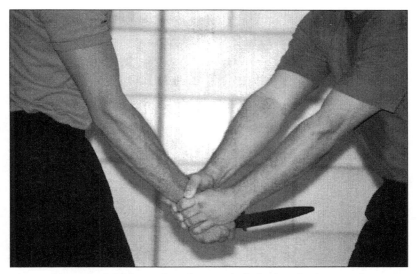

Pictured here, the defender on the right controls the knife with a V-grip technique.

The Bottom Line is...

Regardless of its defensive limitations, the cane is still an invaluable self-defense weapon that can save your life when the chips are down. The important point is to understand some of these inherent limitations and work around them.

Having said that, let's take a look at some of the possible defensive techniques you can perform with the tactical cane.

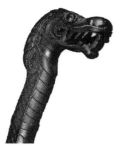

There are a lot of senseis (teachers) out there who are doing a lot more harm than good by making people believe that the cane or walking stick is the be-all and end-all self-defense solution. No self-defense technique, weapon or methodology is an end in itself.

Defensive Cane Techniques

As I stated earlier, a cane or walking stick isn't capable of stopping a vicious compound attack. However, it can be very effective when defending against a single strike.

Defensive cane fighting techniques include blocks, deflections and mobility and footwork. Let's begin with blocking techniques.

High Block

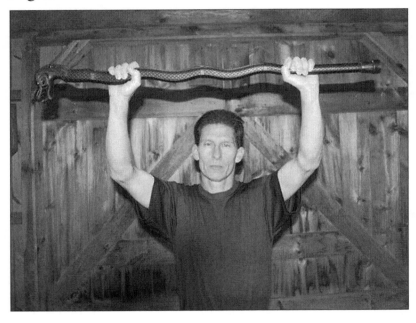

The high block is used to defend against either a powerful bludgeon strike or overhead punch directed at the top section of your head and shoulders.

To perform the block, assume a quarterstaff grip and raise your cane above your head to meet the oncoming blow. Be certain both of your arms are slightly bent.

Right Side Mid-Block

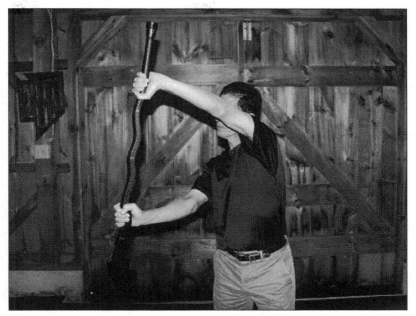

The right side mid-block is used to defend against a powerful bludgeon strike or haymaker punch directed toward the right side of your head, chest and torso.

To perform the block, assume a quarterstaff grip and move your stick across your body to meet the assailant's strike. Again, keep both of your arms slightly bent.

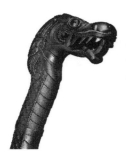

When blocking or deflecting your assailant's blow, be aware of your cane's reverberation path. Stick reverberation occurs when your weapon absorbs the assailant's force, causing it to bounce back at you with significant force.

Left Side Mid-Block

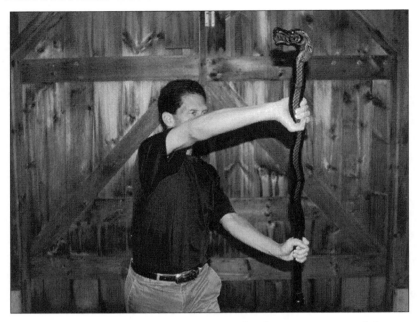

The left side mid-block is used to defend against a powerful bludgeon strike or haymaker punch directed toward the left side of your head, chest and torso.

To perform the block, assume a quarterstaff grip and move your stick across your body to meet the assailant's strike. Again, keep both of your arms slightly bent.

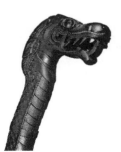

When using a tactical cane as a defensive tool, keep your stick in front of your face and torso at all times. Learn to "hide behind your weapon."

Low Block

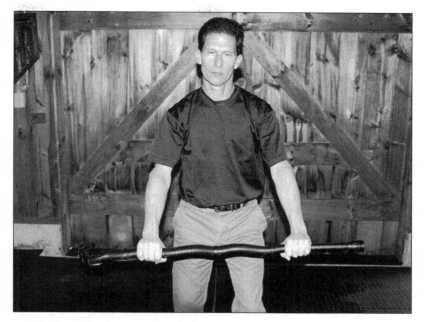

The low block is used to defend against a powerful bludgeon strike or knee or leg strikes directed toward the lower section of your body.

To perform the block, assume a quarterstaff grip and lower your cane to meet the imminent attack. Again, keep both of your arms slightly bent.

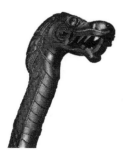

Ideally, your best defense is a strong and powerful offense, but in reality, there will be situations and circumstances that demand a defensive response. However, don't misunderstand the necessity of a strong defense by becoming a defensive fighter.

Cane Deflections

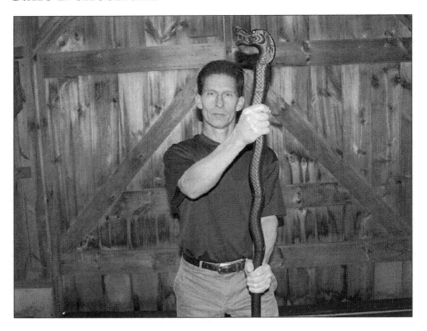

Unlike the block, a cane deflection is used to redirect or deflect your assailant's strike to either the right or left sides of your face or body. Generally, deflections will flow into a counterstrike, and they are commonly used against a linear attack.

To perform the deflection, assume a high point hand grip and move your stick across your body to deflect the assailant's linear strike. Again, remember to keep both of your arms slightly bent when executing the movement.

Deflecting to the Left

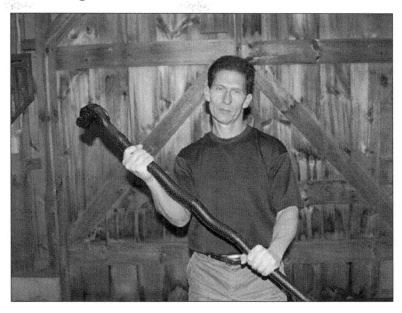

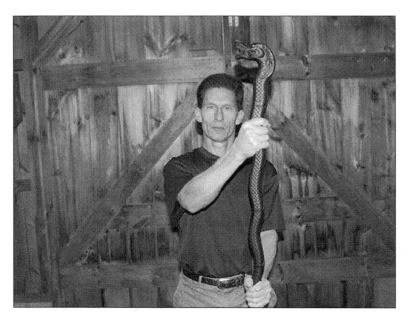

Deflecting to the Right

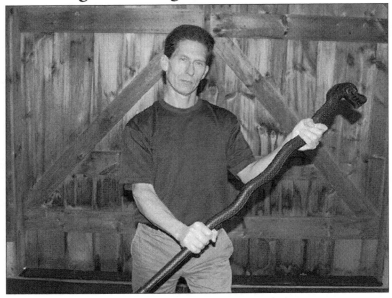

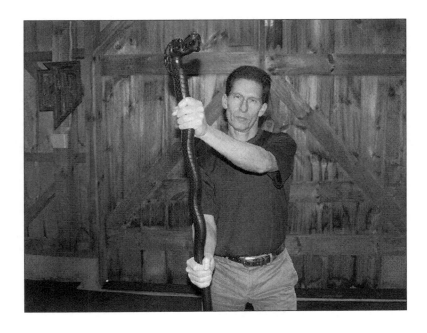

Move While You Defend

The final component of cane defensive skills is mobility and footwork. One of the biggest mistakes you can make when defending with a cane or walking stick is to just stand still and block or deflect the attack. It's of paramount importance to also move when you're defending against an attack.

There are seven strategic reasons why mobility is essential for cane defense. They are:

1. A moving target is harder to hit.

2. Your assailant can misjudge your proximity.

3. It throws the assailant's offensive timing off.

4. It helps prevent multiple attackers from surrounding you.

5. It possible, it helps you locate escape routes.

6. It enhances the overall power of your cane strikes (movement is a natural power generator).

7. Sometimes it can help you acquire a superior position.

Footwork & Mobility

I define mobility as the ability to move your body quickly and freely, which is accomplished through basic footwork. The safest footwork involves quick, economical steps performed on the balls of your feet, while you remain relaxed and balanced. Keep in mind that balance is one of the most important considerations when cane fighting.

Basic footwork can be used for both offensive and defensive purposes, and it is structured around four general directions: forward, backward, right, and left. However, always remember this footwork rule of thumb: *Always move the foot closest to the direction you want to go first, and let the other foot follow an equal distance.*

Cane Fighting

This prevents cross-stepping, which can be disastrous in a high-risk combat situation.

Basic Footwork Movements

1. Moving forward (advance)- from your cane fighting stance, first move your front foot forward (approximately 12 -18 inches) and then move your rear foot an equal distance.

2. Moving backward (retreat) - from your stance, first move your rear foot backward (approximately 12 - 18 inches) and then move your front foot an equal distance.

3. Moving right (sidestep right) - from your stance, first move your right foot to the right (approximately 12 - 18 inches) and then move your left foot an equal distance.

4. Moving left (sidestep left) - from your stance, first move your left foot to the left (approximately 12 - 18 inches) and then move your right foot an equal distance.

Practice these four movements for 10 to 15 minutes a day in front of a full-length mirror. In a couple weeks, your footwork should be quick, balanced, and natural.

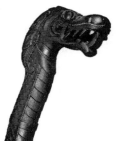

No form of combat (armed or unarmed) is ever going to be a static encounter. There is always going to be some movement during a self-defense encounter. Be prepared for it!

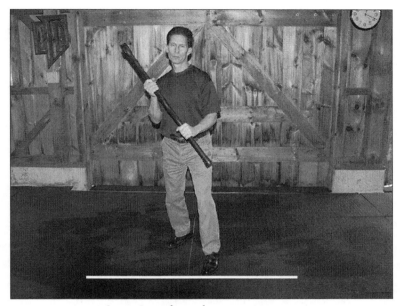

Step 1: Begin from a basic stance position.

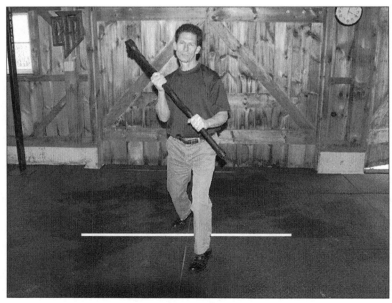

Step 2: Advance forward.

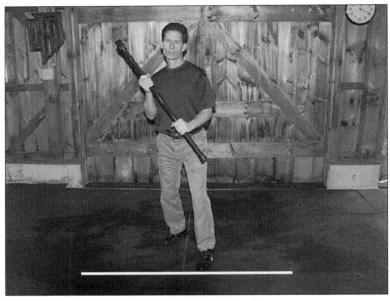

Step 3: Retreat.

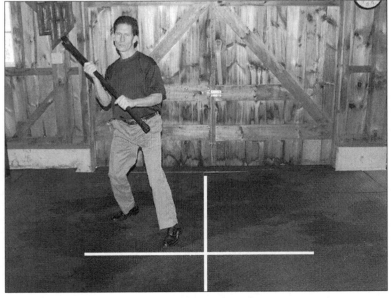

Step 4: Sidestep to the right.

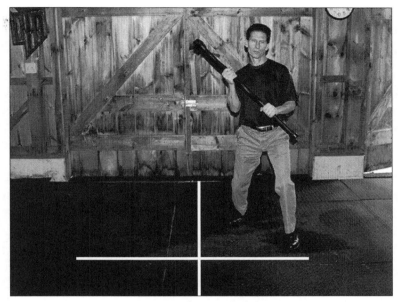

Step 5: Sidestep to the left.

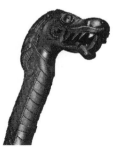

Pushing off the balls of your feet is a critical aspect of an effective offensive attack. However, when moving forward, always keep at least one foot in contact with the ground. You never want to be "airborne" in a fight.

Circling Right and Left

Strategic circling is an advanced form of footwork where you will use your front leg as a pivot point. This type of movement permits you to move 360-degrees around your adversary and also allow you to counterstrike from various angles. Strategic circling can be performed from either a left or right stance.

Circling left (from a left stance) - this means you'll be moving your body around the opponent in a clockwise direction. From a left stance, step 8 to 12 inches to the left with your left foot, then use your left leg as a pivot point and wheel your entire rear leg to the left until the correct stance and positioning is acquired.

Circling right (from a right stance) - from a right stance, step 8 to 12 inches to the right with your right foot, then use your right leg as a pivot point and wheel your entire rear leg to the right until the correct stance and positioning is acquired.

Avoid Cross-Stepping When Defending

Cross-stepping is the process of crossing one foot in front or behind the other when moving around the adversary. Such sloppy footwork makes you vulnerable to a variety of problems. Some include:

- It severely compromises your balance.
- It restricts the offensive flow of attack.
- It limits quick and rapid footwork.
- It can lead to a sprained ankle.

As I said earlier, the best way to avoid cross-stepping is to follow this basic footwork rule of thumb: *Always move the foot closest to the direction you want to go first, and let the other foot follow an equal distance.*

Explosive Footwork

Explosive footwork is another important component of cane fighting. In fact, this type of dynamic movement plays a vital role in both offensive and defensive fighting. In offense, explosive footwork allows you to reach your target and maintain a devastating compound attack. In defense, it permits you to disengage quickly from the range of an overwhelming assault.

Explosive footwork is predicated on the following five important factors. They include the following:

1. **Basic footwork** - you must first master the basic footwork skills before incorporating ballistic movements.

2. **Proper body posture** - maintaining correct body posture through footwork movements will prevent loss of balance.

3. **Powerful legs**- strong and powerful upper and lower legs will allow you to launch your body effortlessly through the ranges of fighting.

4. **Equal weight distribution** - a noncommittal weight distribution (fifty percent on each leg) will permit you to move instantly in any direction.

5. **Raised heel** - this creates a springlike effect in your footwork movements.

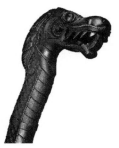

Use the "step and drag" footwork when standing on slippery or unstable terrain. Some examples of unstable terrain include ice, snow, wet grass, wet concrete, wet leaves, wet metal, wet wood, sand, gravel, damp mulch, mud, and rock.

Cane Fighting

Chapter Seven
Cane Fighting Workouts

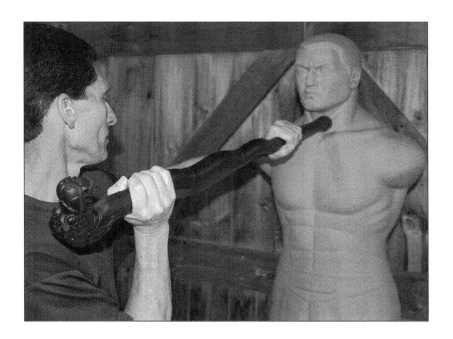

Warming-Up & Stretching Out

Before training, it's important
that you first warm up and
stretch out. Warming up
slowly increases the internal
temperature of your body while
stretching improves your workout
performance, keeps you
flexible, and helps reduce the
possibility of an injury.

Some of the best exercises
for warming up are jumping
jacks, rope skipping or
a short jog before training. Another effective method of warming
up your muscles is to perform light and easy movements with the
weights.

When stretching out, keep in mind that all movements should be
performed in a slow and controlled manner. Try to hold your stretch
for a minimum of sixty seconds and avoid all bouncing movements.
You should feel mild tension on the muscle that is being stretched.
Remember to stay relaxed and focus on what you are doing. Here are
seven stretches that should be performed.

Neck stretch - from a comfortable standing position, slowly tilt
your head to the right side of your neck, holding it for a count of
twenty. Then tilt your head to the left side for approximately twenty
seconds. Stretch each side of the neck at least three times.

Triceps stretch - from a standing position, keep your knees
slightly bent, extend your right arm overhead, hold the elbow of your
right arm with your left hand, and slowly pull your right elbow to
the left. Keep your hips straight as you stretch your triceps gently for

thirty seconds. Repeat this stretch for the other arm.

Hamstring stretch - from a seated position on the floor, extend your right leg in front of you with your toe pointing to the ceiling. Place the sole of your left foot in the inside of your extended leg. Gently lean forward at the hips and stretch out the hamstrings of your right leg. Hold this position for a minimum of sixty seconds. Switch legs and repeat the stretch.

Spinal twist - from a seated position on the floor, extend your right leg in front of you. Raise your left leg and place it to the outside of your right leg. Place your right elbow on the outside of your left thigh. Stabilize your stretch with your elbow and twist your upper body and head to your left side. Breathe naturally and hold this stretch for a minimum of thirty seconds. Switch legs and repeat this stretch for the other side.

Quad stretch - assume a sitting position on the floor with your hamstrings folded and resting on top of your calves. Your toes should be pointed behind you, and your instep should be flush with the ground. Sit comfortably into the stretch and hold for a minimum of sixty seconds.

Prone stretch - lay on the ground with your back to the floor. Exhale as you straighten your arms and legs. Your fingers and toes should be stretching in opposite directions. Hold this stretch for thirty seconds.

Groin stretch - sit on the ground with the soles of your feet touching each other. Grab hold of your feet and slowly pull yourself forward until mild tension is felt in your groin region. Hold this position for a minimum of sixty seconds.

Cane Twists

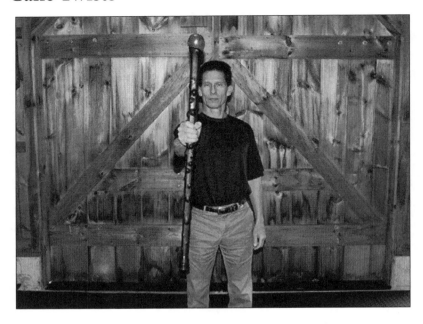

Cane twisting is great for warming up and strengthening your hands, wrists and forearms for the rigors of cane fighting. Remember to always start off slowly and progressively increase the duration of the exercise.

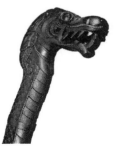

Because of the weight of the stick, cane twisting is very taxing on the muscles and tendons of the wrist and forearms. Remember to take your time when performing this exercise for the very first time.

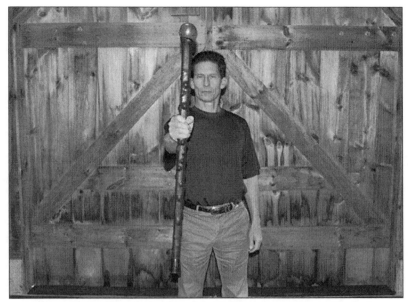

Step 1: With your right hand, grab hold of the center portion of the shaft.

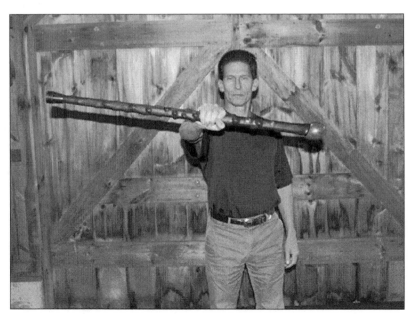

Step 2: With your arm extended in front of you, rotate the cane to your left.

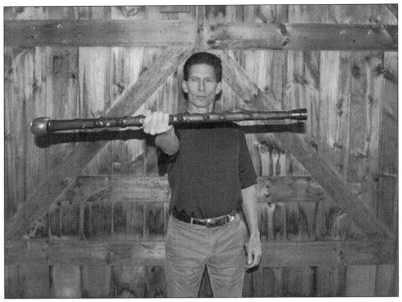

Step 3: Rotate the cane 180 degrees to the right.

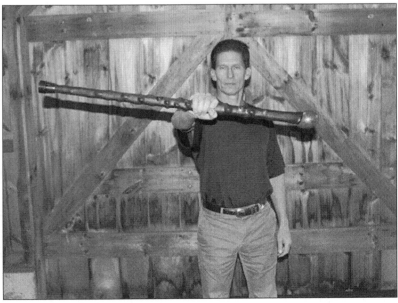

Step 4: Continue rotating your cane back and forth for a duration of thirty seconds.

164

Cane Twirls

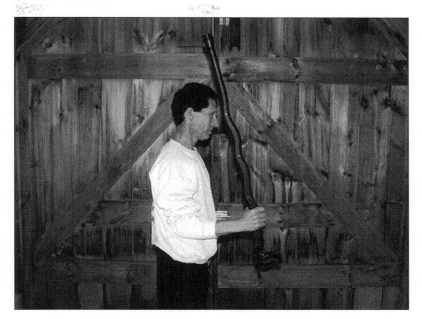

The cane twirl is an excellent strengthening and dexterity exercise that should be practiced on a regular basis. This is especially taxing on the wrists, so remember to start slowly and progressively increase the speed of the movement.

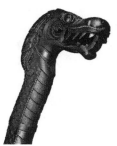

If you initially discover that your cane is too heavy or cumbersome to twirl, consider first practicing with a 26-inch rattan stick.

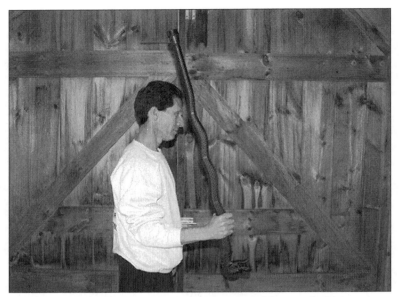

Step 1: With your right hand, hold the lower portion of the cane shaft between your thumb and index finger.

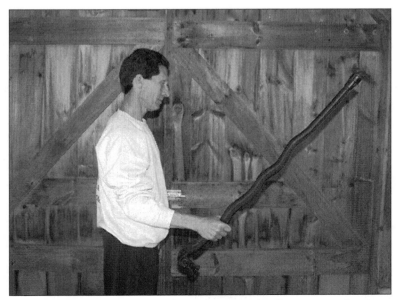

Step 2: Forcefully spin the weapon forward at your side, allowing your other three fingers to move freely.

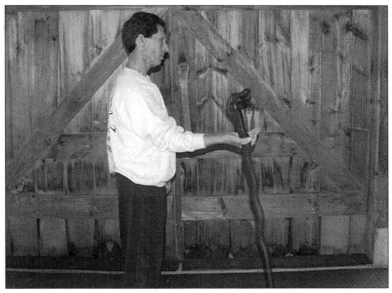

Step 3: When correctly done, the cane should twirl 360 degrees.

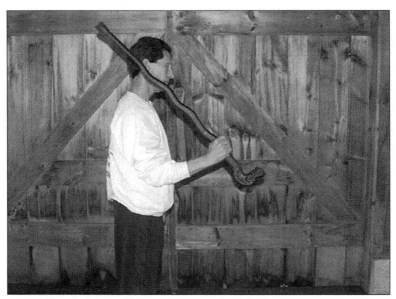

Step 4: Continue twirling the stick in a smooth and controlled manner for a duration of 30 to 60 seconds. Switch and perform the exercise with your left hand.

Cane Fighting on the Body Opponent Bag

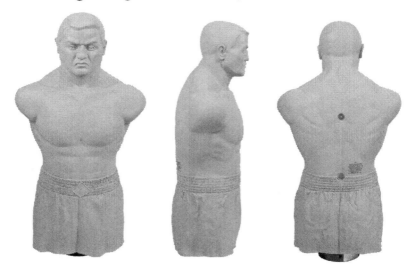

As I discussed in Chapter 4, the body opponent bag is one of the best tools for developing striking proficiency with the tactical cane. Unlike the traditional heavy bag, this freestanding mannequin bag provides realistic life-like targets that you can attack with full-speed, full-force cane strikes.

Effective cane fighting skills take time and practice to master. Remember to start out slowly and progressively build up the speed and intensity of your strikes. If you are a beginner, avoid the urge to attack the bag with maximum speed and force. Take your time and enjoy the process of learning a new fighting skill.

Also, one of the biggest mistakes you can make when working out on the body opponent bag is to stand still and strike the bag. Cane targets are located on all four sides of the bag, so you should take full advantage by moving around it when training.

Finally, before you begin any workout program, including those suggested in this chapter, it's important to check with your physician to see whether you have any condition that might be aggravated by strenuous exercise.

Body Opponent Bag Schematics

Here, I'm going to provide you with a variety of schematics that will allow you to practice cane fighting combinations on your own. These diagrams are just examples of what you can do, remember you are only limited by your imagination. However, keep in mind that your striking combinations must also be logical and predicated on the probable reaction dynamics of a real opponent.

How to Use the Schematics

These striking schematics are designed to give you a clear visual reference point of how each cane strike flows into the next. The numbers on the body opponent bag **do not** represent the angle of attack, but rather the sequence or order of each hit.

To get you started, I have included several photographs demonstrating how the schematics translate into actual cane fighting techniques applied on the body opponent bag.

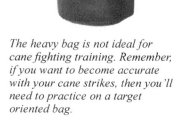

The heavy bag is not ideal for cane fighting training. Remember, if you want to become accurate with your cane strikes, then you'll need to practice on a target oriented bag.

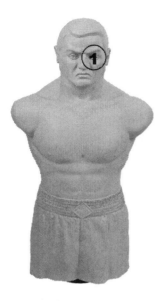

Cane Strikes

1. Angle 7

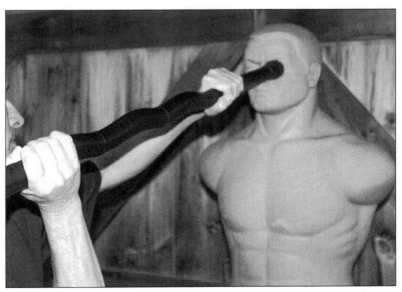

Here, the practitioner demonstrates how the schematic translates to an actual technique executed on the body opponent bag. In this instance, number one represents an angle 7 thrust to the eye.

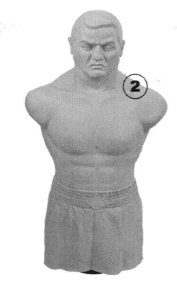

Cane Strikes

1. Angle 7

2. **Angle 1**

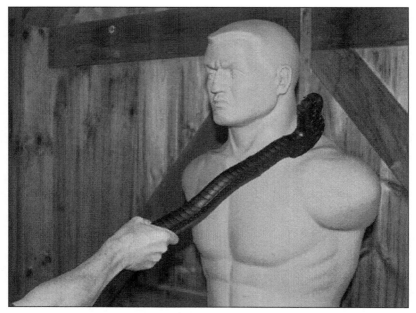

The second technique is a diagonal cane strike to the collarbone (angle 1).

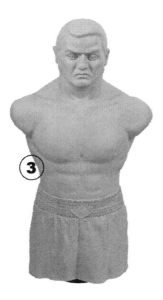

Cane Strikes

1. Angle 7
2. Angle 1
3. **Angle 4**

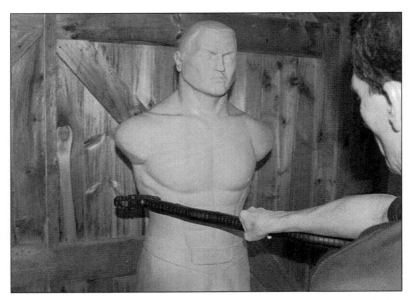

The third technique in the sequence is a horizontal cane strike to the ribs (angle 4).

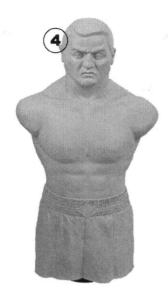

Cane Strikes

1. Angle 7
2. Angle 1
3. Angle 4
4. **Angle 2**

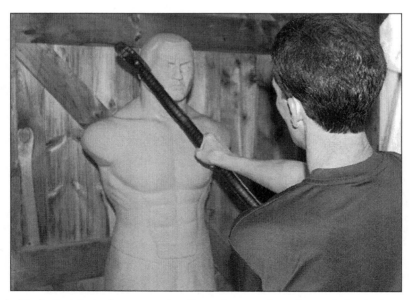

The forth strike in the sequence is a diagonal cane strike to the temple (angle 2).

The Nine Striking Angles

For your convenience, I've included a quick review of the nine angles of attack that will help you quickly identify the correct striking angle in the sequence without having to go back to chapter five. However, if you would like more detailed information about the nine angles of attack, please refer to that chapter.

Angle 1

Angle One is a diagonal forehand strike traveling from right to left. Impact can be made with the handle, knob, or shaft of your cane. Anatomical targets include your assailant's temple, clavicle, back of neck, spine, elbow, ribs, thigh, knee joint, shins, and hands.

Angle 2

Angle Two is a diagonal backhand strike traveling from left to right. Impact can be made with the handle, knob, or shaft of your cane. Anatomical targets include your assailant's temple, clavicle, back of neck, spine, elbow, ribs, thigh, knee joint, shins, and hands.

Angle 3

Angle Three is a horizontal forehand strike traveling from right to left. Impact can be made with the handle, knob, or shaft of your cane. Anatomical targets include your assailant's temple, back of neck, spine, elbow, ribs, thigh, shins, knee joint, and hands.

Angle 4

Angle Four is a horizontal backhand strike traveling from left to right. Impact is made with either the handle, knob, or shaft of your cane. Anatomical targets include your assailant's temple, back of neck, spine, elbow, ribs, thigh, shins, knee joint, and hands.

Angle 5

Angle Five is an upward diagonal forehand moving from right to left. Impact is made with either the handle, knob, or shaft of your cane. Anatomical targets include your assailant's temple, chin, elbow, ribs, thigh, shins, knee joint, and hands.

Angle 6

Angle Six is an upward diagonal backhand strike moving from left to right. Impact is made with either the handle, knob, or shaft of your cane. Anatomical targets include your assailant's temple, chin, elbow, ribs, thigh, shins, knee joint, and hands.

Angle 7

Angle Seven is a linear thrust delivered anywhere on the assailant's centerline. Impact is made with tip of your cane. Anatomical targets include your assailant's face, eyes, throat, solar plexus, spine, back of neck, and groin.

Angle 8

Angle Eight is a downward vertical strike. Impact is made with either the handle, knob, shaft or tip of your cane. Anatomical targets include your assailant's head, clavicle, back of neck, spine, elbow, ribs, thigh, knee joint, and hands.

Angle 9

Angle Nine is an upward vertical strike. Impact is made with either the handle, knob, or shaft of your cane. Anatomical targets include your assailant's chin, elbow, ribs, groin, thigh, knee joint, and hands.

Cane Striking Combinations (Front Targets)

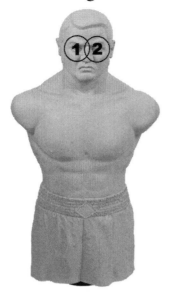

Combination #1

1. Angle 7 thrust
2. Angle 7 thrust

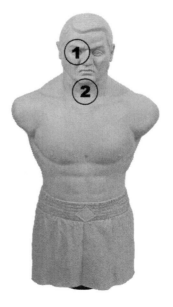

Combination #2

1. Angle 7 thrust
2. Angle 9 strike

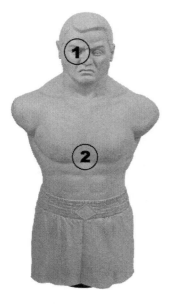

Combination #3

1. Angle 7 thrust
2. Angle 7 thrust

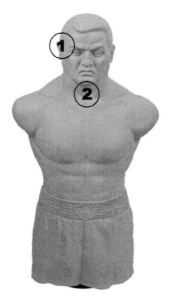

Combination #4

1. Angle 2 strike
2. Angle 7 thrust

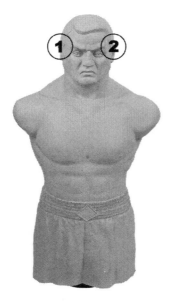

Combination #5

1. Angle 4 strike
2. Angle 3 strike

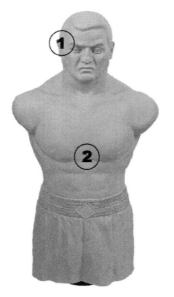

Combination #6

1. Angle 2 strike
2. Angle 7 thrust

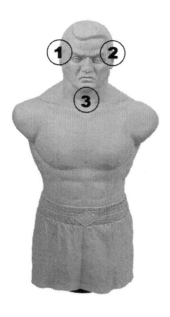

Combination #7

1. Angle 2 strike
2. Angle 1 strike
3. Angle 7 thrust

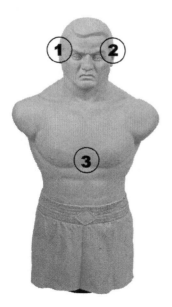

Combination #8

1. Angle 2 strike
2. Angle 1 strike
3. Angle 7 thrust

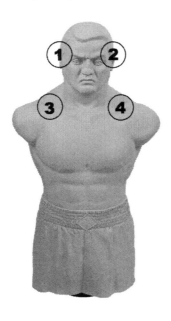

Combination #9

1. Angle 3 strike
2. Angle 4 strike
3. Angle 2 strike
4. Angle 1 strike

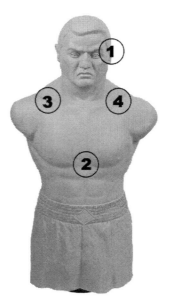

Combination #10

1. Angle 1 strike
2. Angle 7 thrust
3. Angle 2 strike
4. Angle 1 strike

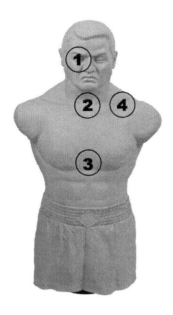

Combination #11

1. Angle 7 thrust
2. Angle 7 thrust
3. Angle 7 thrust
4. Angle 8 strike

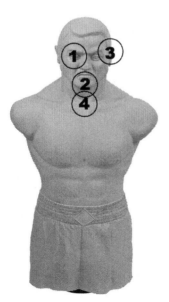

Combination #12

1. Angle 7 thrust
2. Angle 9 strike
3. Angle 1 strike
4. Angle 7 thrust

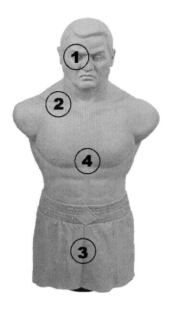

Combination #13

1. Angle 7 thrust
2. Angle 2 strike
3. Angle 7 thrust
4. Angle 9 strike

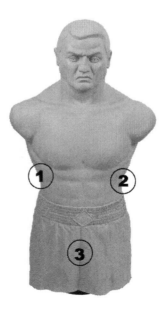

Combination #14

1. Angle 6 strike
2. Angle 5 strike
3. Angle 7 thrust

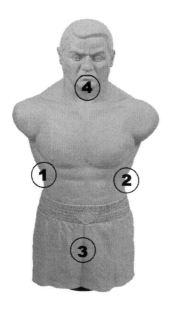

Combination #15

1. Angle 4 strike
2. Angle 3 strike
3. Angle 7 thrust
4. Angle 9 strike

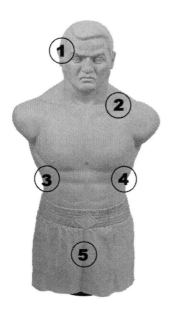

Combination #16

1. Angle 2 strike
2. Angle 1 strike
3. Angle 4 strike
4. Angle 3 strike
5. Angle 7 thrust

Cane Striking Combinations (Rear Targets)

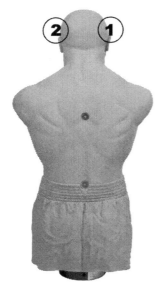

Combination #17

1. Angle 1 strike
2. Angle 2 strike

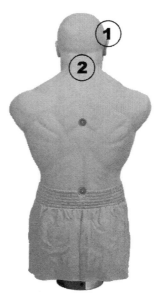

Combination #18

1. Angle 1 strike
2. Angle 7 thrust

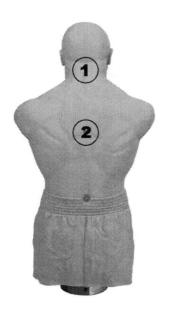

Combination #19

1. Angle 8 strike
2. Angle 7 thrust

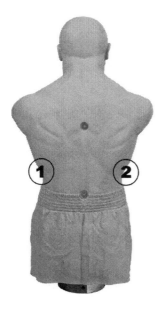

Combination #20

1. Angle 4 strike
2. Angle 3 strike

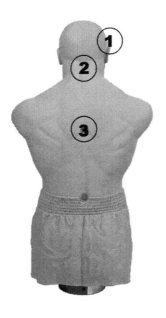

Combination #21

1. Angle 1 strike
2. Angle 8 strike
3. Angle 7 thrust

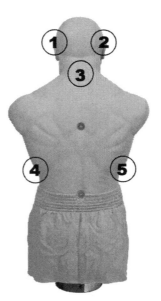

Combination #22

1. Angle 2 strike
2. Angle 1 strike
3. Angle 7 thrust
4. Angle 4 strike
5. Angle 3 strike

Cane Striking Combinations (Side Targets)

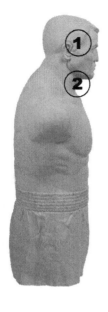

Combination #23

1. Angle 7 thrust
2. Angle 5 strike

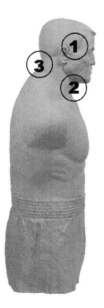

Combination #24

1. Angle 7 thrust
2. Angle 5 strike
3. Angle 2 strike

187

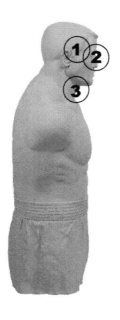

Combination #25

1. Angle 7 thrust
2. Angle 1 strike
3. Angle 5 strike

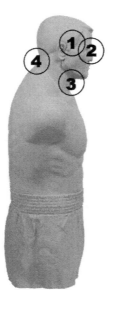

Combination #26

1. Angle 7 thrust
2. Angle 1 strike
3. Angle 5 strike
4. Angle 2 strike

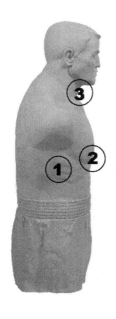

Combination #27

1. Angle 7 thrust
2. Angle 3 strike
3. Angle 5 strike

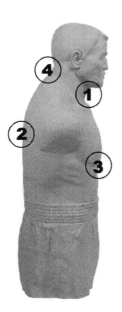

Combination #28

1. Angle 5 strike
2. Angle 4 strike
3. Angle 3 strike
4. Angle 2 strike

Three Training Methods for Cane Fighting

Over the past thirty years of teaching the martial arts, I have developed three unique training methodologies you cane apply to cane fighting on the body opponent bag. They include Proficiency, Conditioning and Street Training. Let's take a look at each one.

Conditioning Training

Conditioning Training is used by individuals who wish to train on the body opponent bag for specified period of time called *rounds*. Depending on the practitioner's level of conditioning, each round can range anywhere from one to five minutes. Each round is then separated by either 30-second, one-minute or two-minute breaks. A good cane fighting workout consists of at least five rounds.

Conditioning Training is performed at a moderate pace, and it develops cardiovascular fitness, muscular endurance, fluidity, rhythm, distancing, timing, speed, footwork, and balance.

Most importantly, Conditioning Training requires that you have a fundamental understanding of combining cane strikes together into logical combinations.

Proficiency Training

The second training methodology is Proficiency Training, and it's generally used people who want to sharpen one specific cane strike at a time by executing it over and over for a prescribed number of repetitions. Each time the technique is performed with "clean" form at various speeds. Cane strikes are also performed with the eyes closed to develop a kinesthetic "feel" for the action.

Proficiency Training on the body opponent bag develops speed, power, accuracy, non-telegraphic movement, balance, and general psychomotor skill.

Street Training

The third and final training methodology is Street Training, and it's specially designed for real world self-defense preparation.

Since most self-defense altercations are explosive, lasting an average of 20 seconds, the practitioner must prepare for this possible scenario. This means delivering powerful cane fighting combinations with vicious intent for approximately 20 seconds, resting one minute, and then repeating the process.

Street Training prepares you for the stress and immediate fatigue of a real fight. It also develops speed, power, explosiveness, target selection and recognition, timing, footwork and breath control.

Designing Your Cane Fighting Workout

While all three training methodologies are important, we are going to focus exclusively on Conditioning Training, which means we are going to focus on "time-based" workouts.

Time-Based Workouts

Essentially, a time-based cane fighting workout is based on "rounds" and it's an ideal way to structure your workouts. Before you begin, now is the time to decide on the duration of your rounds as well as the rest intervals.

In most cases, experienced practitioners will work the body opponent bag for three-minute rounds with one-minute rest periods. Depending on their level of conditioning and specific training goals, they might do this for a total of 5 to 8 rounds.

Cane Fighting

Initially, you'll need to experiment with both the round duration and rest intervals to see what works best for you. Remember to start off slow and progressively build up the intensity and length of your workouts. Don't forget to work with the bag and not try to kill it!

To get you started, here are some time-based cane fighting workouts you might want to try. Keep in mind, the advanced level workouts are for experienced practitioners who have a minimum of five years of cane fighting training.

Time-Based Cane Fighting Workouts			
Skill Level	Duration of Each Round	Rest Period	Total Number of rounds
Beginner	1 minute	2 minutes	3
Beginner	1 minute	1 minute	3
Beginner	2 minutes	2 minutes	3
Beginner	2 minutes	1 minute	3
Intermediate	3 minutes	2 minutes	5
Intermediate	3 minutes	1 minute	5
Intermediate	3 minutes	2 minutes	6
Intermediate	3 minutes	1 minute	6
Advanced	4 minutes	2 minutes	8
Advanced	4 minutes	1 minute	8
Advanced	5 minutes	2 minutes	10
Advanced	5 minutes	1 minute	10

Conditioning and Strength Training

One of the most important and often neglected aspects of cane fighting is conditioning and strength training. It's no surprise that strong hands, wrists, and forearms will significantly enhance your fighting skills.

In fact, powerful hands and forearms will amplify the power of your strikes and significantly improve your weapon retention. Strong forearms will also help minimize premature fatigue when working out. Fortunately, there are several effective hand and forearm exercises you can perform to strengthen these muscles. Let's take a look at some of them.

Power Putty

One excellent hand exerciser that strengthens all the muscles in your fingers and hands is Power Putty. Essentially, Power Putty is a flexible silicone rubber that can be squeezed, stretched, and crushed. Begin using the putty for ten-minute sessions and progressively build up to thirty minutes. Remember to work both hands equally.

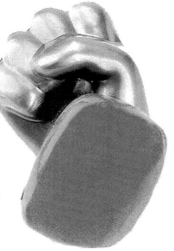

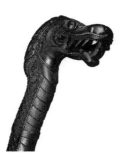

Power putty is sold in a variety of different resistance levels ranging from extra soft to firm.

Hand Grippers

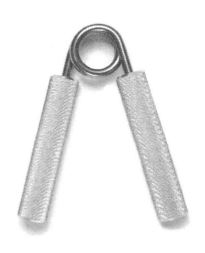

Another effective way to strengthen your hands, wrists and forearms is to work out with heavy duty hand grippers. While there is a big selection of them on the market, I prefer using the Captains of Crush brand. These high-quality grippers are virtually indestructible and they are sold in a variety of different resistance levels ranging from 60 to 365 pounds.

Weight Training

Finally, you can also condition your wrists and forearms by performing various forearm exercises with free weights. Exercises like hammer curls, reverse curls, wrist curls, and reverse wrist curls are excellent for developing powerful forearms. When training your forearms, be sure to work both your extensor and flexor muscles. Let's look at some of the exercises.

Barbell Wrist Curls

This exercise strengthens the flexor muscles. Perform five sets of 8-10 repetitions. To perform the exercise, follow these steps:

1. Sit at the end of a bench, grab a barbell with an underhand grip and place both of your hands close together.

2. In a smooth and controlled fashion, slowly bend your wrists and lower the barbell toward the floor.

3. Contract your forearms and curl the weight back to the starting position.

Reverse Wrist Curls

This exercise develops and strengthens the extensor muscle of the forearm. Perform six sets of 6-8 repetitions. To perform the exercise, follow these steps:

1. Sit at the end of a bench, hold a barbell with an overhand grip (your hands should be approximately 11 inches apart) and place your forearms on top of your thighs.

2. Slowly lower the barbell as far as your wrists will allow.

3. Flex your wrists upward back to the starting position.

Behind-the-Back Wrist Curls

This exercise strengthens both the flexor muscles of the forearms. Perform five sets of 6-8 repetitions To perform the exercise, follow these steps:

1. Hold a barbell behind your back at arm's length (your hands should be approximately shoulder-width apart).

2. Uncurl your finger and let the barbell slowly roll down your palms.

3. Close your hands and roll the barbell back into your hands.

Hammer Curls

This exercise strengthens both the Brachialis and Brachioradialis muscles. Perform five sets of 8-10 repetitions. To perform the exercise, follow these steps:

1. Stand with both feet approximately shoulder-width apart, with both dumbbells at your sides.

2. Keeping your elbows close to your body and your palms facing inward, slowly curl both dumbbells upward towards your shoulders.

195

3. Slowly return to the starting position.

Reverse Barbell Curls

Reverse curls can be a great alternative to hammer curls. This exercise strengthens both the Brachialis and Brachioradialis muscles. Perform five sets of 8-10 repetitions. To perform the exercise, follow these steps:

1. Stand with both feet approximately shoulder width apart. Hold a barbell with your palms facing down (pronated grip).

2. Keeping your upper arms stationary, curl the weights up until the bar is at shoulder level.

3. Slowly return to the starting position.

Glossary

A

accuracy—The precise or exact projection of force. Accuracy is also defined as the ability to execute a combative movement with precision and exactness.

adaptability—The ability to physically and psychologically adjust to new or different conditions or circumstances of combat.

advanced first-strike tools—Offensive techniques that are specifically used when confronted with multiple opponents.

aerobic exercise—Literally, "with air." Exercise that elevates the heart rate to a training level for a prolonged period of time, usually 30 minutes.

affective preparedness – One of the three components of preparedness. Affective preparedness means being emotionally, philosophically, and spiritually prepared for the strains of combat. See cognitive preparedness and psychomotor preparedness.

aggression—Hostile and injurious behavior directed toward a person.

aggressive response—One of the three possible counters when assaulted by a grab, choke, or hold from a standing position. Aggressive response requires you to counter the enemy with destructive blows and strikes. See moderate response and passive response.

aggressive hand positioning—Placement of hands so as to imply aggressive or hostile intentions.

agility—An attribute of combat. One's ability to move his or her

Cane Fighting

body quickly and gracefully.

amalgamation—A scientific process of uniting or merging.

ambidextrous—The ability to perform with equal facility on both the right and left sides of the body.

anabolic steroids – synthetic chemical compounds that resemble the male sex hormone testosterone. This performance-enhancing drug is known to increase lean muscle mass, strength, and endurance.

analysis and integration—One of the five elements of CFA's mental component. This is the painstaking process of breaking down various elements, concepts, sciences, and disciplines into their atomic parts, and then methodically and strategically analyzing, experimenting, and drastically modifying the information so that it fulfills three combative requirements: efficiency, effectiveness, and safety. Only then is it finally integrated into the CFA system.

anatomical striking targets—The various anatomical body targets that can be struck and which are especially vulnerable to potential harm. They include: the eyes, temple, nose, chin, back of neck, front of neck, solar plexus, ribs, groin, thighs, knees, shins, and instep.

anchoring – The strategic process of trapping the assailant's neck or limb in order to control the range of engagement during razing.

assailant—A person who threatens or attacks another person.

assault—The threat or willful attempt to inflict injury upon the person of another.

assault and battery—The unlawful touching of another person without justification.

assessment—The process of rapidly gathering, analyzing, and accurately evaluating information in terms of threat and danger. You can assess people, places, actions, and objects.

attack—Offensive action designed to physically control, injure, or kill another person.

attitude—One of the three factors that determine who wins a street fight. Attitude means being emotionally, philosophically, and spiritually liberated from societal and religious mores. See skills and knowledge.

attributes of combat—The physical, mental, and spiritual qualities that enhance combat skills and tactics.

awareness—Perception or knowledge of people, places, actions, and objects. (In CFA, there are three categories of tactical awareness: criminal awareness, situational awareness, and self-awareness.)

B

balance—One's ability to maintain equilibrium while stationary or moving.

blading the body—Strategically positioning your body at a 45-degree angle.

blitz and disengage—A style of sparring whereby a fighter moves into a range of combat, unleashes a strategic compound attack, and then quickly disengages to a safe distance. Of all sparring methodologies, the blitz and disengage most closely resembles a real street fight.

block—A defensive tool designed to intercept the assailant's attack by placing a non-vital target between the assailant's strike and your vital body target.

body composition—The ratio of fat to lean body tissue.

body language—Nonverbal communication through posture, gestures, and facial expressions.

body mechanics—Technically precise body movement during the execution of a body weapon, defensive technique, or other fighting maneuver.

body tackle – A tackle that occurs when your opponent haphazardly rushes forward and plows his body into yours.

body weapon—Also known as a tool, one of the various body parts that can be used to strike or otherwise injure or kill a criminal assailant.

burn out—A negative emotional state acquired by physically over- training. Some symptoms include: illness, boredom, anxiety, disinterest in training, and general sluggishness.

C

cadence—Coordinating tempo and rhythm to establish a timing pattern of movement.

cardiorespiratory conditioning—The component of physical fitness that deals with the heart, lungs, and circulatory system.

centerline—An imaginary vertical line that divides your body in half and which contains many of your vital anatomical targets.

choke holds—Holds that impair the flow of blood or oxygen to the brain.

circular movements—Movements that follow the direction of a curve.

close-quarter combat—One of the three ranges of knife and bludgeon combat. At this distance, you can strike, slash, or stab your assailant with a variety of close-quarter techniques.

cognitive development—One of the five elements of CFA's mental component. The process of developing and enhancing your fighting skills through specific mental exercises and techniques. See analysis and integration, killer instinct, philosophy, and strategic/tactical development.

cognitive exercises—Various mental exercises used to enhance fighting skills and tactics.

cognitive preparedness – One of the three components of preparedness. Cognitive preparedness means being equipped with the strategic concepts, principles, and general knowledge of combat. See affective preparedness and psychomotor preparedness.

combat-oriented training—Training that is specifically related to the harsh realities of both armed and unarmed combat. See ritual-oriented training and sport-oriented training.

combative arts—The various arts of war. See martial arts.

combative attributes—See attributes of combat.

combative fitness—A state characterized by cardiorespiratory and muscular/skeletal conditioning, as well as proper body composition.

combative mentality—Also known as the killer instinct, this is a combative state of mind necessary for fighting. See killer instinct.

combat ranges—The various ranges of unarmed combat.

combative utility—The quality of condition of being combatively useful.

combination(s)—See compound attack.

common peroneal nerve—A pressure point area located approximately four to six inches above the knee on the midline of the outside of the thigh.

composure—A combative attribute. Composure is a quiet and focused mind-set that enables you to acquire your combative agenda.

compound attack—One of the five conventional methods of attack. Two or more body weapons launched in strategic succession whereby the fighter overwhelms his assailant with a flurry of full speed, full-force blows.

conditioning training—A CFA training methodology requiring the practitioner to deliver a variety of offensive and defensive combinations for a 4-minute period. See proficiency training and street training.

contact evasion—Physically moving or manipulating your body to avoid being tackled by the adversary.

Contemporary Fighting Arts—A modern martial art and self-defense system made up of three parts: physical, mental, and spiritual.

conventional ground-fighting tools—Specific ground-fighting techniques designed to control, restrain, and temporarily incapacitate your adversary. Some conventional ground fighting tactics include: submission holds, locks, certain choking techniques, and specific striking techniques.

coordination—A physical attribute characterized by the ability to perform a technique or movement with efficiency, balance, and accuracy.

counterattack—Offensive action made to counter an assailant's initial attack.

courage—A combative attribute. The state of mind and spirit that enables a fighter to face danger and vicissitudes with confidence, resolution, and bravery.

creatine monohydrate—A tasteless and odorless white powder that mimics some of the effects of anabolic steroids. Creatine is a safe body-building product that can benefit anyone who wants to increase their strength, endurance, and lean muscle mass.

criminal awareness—One of the three categories of CFA awareness. It involves a general understanding and knowledge of the nature and dynamics of a criminal's motivations, mentalities, methods, and capabilities to perpetrate violent crime. See situational awareness and self-awareness.

criminal justice—The study of criminal law and the procedures associated with its enforcement.

criminology—The scientific study of crime and criminals.

cross-stepping—The process of crossing one foot in front of or behind the other when moving.

crushing tactics—Nuclear grappling-range techniques designed to crush the assailant's anatomical targets.

cue word - a unique word or personal statement that helps focus your attention on the execution of a skill, instead of its outcome.

D

deadly force—Weapons or techniques that may result in unconsciousness, permanent disfigurement, or death.

deception—A combative attribute. A stratagem whereby you delude your assailant.

decisiveness—A combative attribute. The ability to follow a tactical course of action that is unwavering and focused.

defense—The ability to strategically thwart an assailant's attack (armed or unarmed).

defensive flow—A progression of continuous defensive responses.

defensive mentality—A defensive mind-set.

defensive reaction time—The elapsed time between an assailant's physical attack and your defensive response to that attack. See offensive reaction time.

demeanor—A person's outward behavior. One of the essential factors to consider when assessing a threatening individual.

diet—A lifestyle of healthy eating.

disingenuous vocalization—The strategic and deceptive

utilization of words to successfully launch a preemptive strike at your adversary.

distancing—The ability to quickly understand spatial relationships and how they relate to combat.

distractionary tactics—Various verbal and physical tactics designed to distract your adversary.

double end bag—A small bag hung from the ceiling and anchored to the floor with two elastic cords. This unique training bag develops striking accuracy, speed, fighting rhythm, timing, eye-hand coordination, footwork and overall defensive skills.

double-leg takedown—A takedown that occurs when your opponent shoots for both of your legs to force you to the ground.

E

ectomorph—One of the three somatotypes. A body type characterized by a high degree of slenderness, angularity, and fragility. See endomorph and mesomorph.

effectiveness—One of the three criteria for a CFA body weapon, technique, tactic, or maneuver. It means the ability to produce a desired effect. See efficiency and safety.

efficiency—One of the three criteria for a CFA body weapon, technique, tactic, or maneuver. It means the ability to reach an objective quickly and economically. See effectiveness and safety.

emotionless—A combative attribute. Being temporarily devoid of human feeling.

endomorph—One of the three somatotypes. A body type characterized by a high degree of roundness, softness, and body fat. See ectomorph and mesomorph.

evasion—A defensive maneuver that allows you to strategically maneuver your body away from the assailant's strike.

evasive sidestepping—Evasive footwork where the practitioner moves to either the right or left side.

evasiveness—A combative attribute. The ability to avoid threat or danger.

excessive force—An amount of force that exceeds the need for a particular event and is unjustified in the eyes of the law.

experimentation—The painstaking process of testing a combative hypothesis or theory.

explosiveness—A combative attribute that is characterized by a sudden outburst of violent energy.

F

fear—A strong and unpleasant emotion caused by the anticipation or awareness of threat or danger. There are three stages of fear in order of intensity: fright, panic, and terror. See fright, panic, and terror.

feeder—A skilled technician who manipulates the focus mitts.

femoral nerve—A pressure point area located approximately 6 inches above the knee on the inside of the thigh.

fighting stance—Any one of the stances used in CFA's system. A strategic posture you can assume when face-to-face with an unarmed assailant(s). The fighting stance is generally used after you have launched your first-strike tool.

fight-or-flight syndrome—A response of the sympathetic nervous system to a fearful and threatening situation, during which it prepares your body to either fight or flee from the perceived danger.

finesse—A combative attribute. The ability to skillfully execute a

Cane Fighting

movement or a series of movements with grace and refinement.

first strike—Proactive force used to interrupt the initial stages of an assault before it becomes a self-defense situation.

first-strike principle—A CFA principle that states that when physical danger is imminent and you have no other tactical option but to fight back, you should strike first, strike fast, and strike with authority and keep the pressure on.

first-strike stance—One of the stances used in CFA's system. A strategic posture used prior to initiating a first strike.

first-strike tools—Specific offensive tools designed to initiate a preemptive strike against your adversary.

fisted blows – Hand blows delivered with a clenched fist.

five tactical options – The five strategic responses you can make in a self-defense situation, listed in order of increasing level of resistance: comply, escape, de-escalate, assert, and fight back.

flexibility—The muscles' ability to move through maximum natural ranges. See muscular/skeletal conditioning.

focus mitts—Durable leather hand mitts used to develop and sharpen offensive and defensive skills.

footwork—Quick, economical steps performed on the balls of the feet while you are relaxed, alert, and balanced. Footwork is structured around four general movements: forward, backward, right, and left.

fractal tool—Offensive or defensive tools that can be used in more than one combat range.

fright—The first stage of fear; quick and sudden fear. See panic and terror.

full Beat – One of the four beat classifications in the Widow Maker Program. The full beat strike has a complete initiation and retraction phase.

G

going postal - a slang term referring to a person who suddenly and unexpectedly attacks you with an explosive and frenzied flurry of blows. Also known as postal attack.

grappling range—One of the three ranges of unarmed combat. Grappling range is the closest distance of unarmed combat from which you can employ a wide variety of close-quarter tools and techniques. The grappling range of unarmed combat is also divided into two planes: vertical (standing) and horizontal (ground fighting). See kicking range and punching range.

grappling-range tools—The various body tools and techniques that are employed in the grappling range of unarmed combat, including head butts; biting, tearing, clawing, crushing, and gouging tactics; foot stomps, horizontal, vertical, and diagonal elbow strikes, vertical and diagonal knee strikes, chokes, strangles, joint locks, and holds. See punching range tools and kicking range tools.

ground fighting—Also known as the horizontal grappling plane, this is fighting that takes place on the ground.

guard—Also known as the hand guard, this refers to a fighter's hand positioning.

guard position—Also known as leg guard or scissors hold, this is a ground-fighting position in which a fighter is on his back holding his opponent between his legs.

H

half beat – One of the four beat classifications in the Widow Maker Program. The half beat strike is delivered through the retraction phase of the proceeding strike.

hand positioning—See guard.

hand wraps—Long strips of cotton that are wrapped around the hands and wrists for greater protection.

haymaker—A wild and telegraphed swing of the arms executed by an unskilled fighter.

head-hunter—A fighter who primarily attacks the head.

heavy bag—A large cylindrical bag used to develop kicking, punching, or striking power.

high-line kick—One of the two different classifications of a kick. A kick that is directed to targets above an assailant's waist level. See low-line kick.

hip fusing—A full-contact drill that teaches a fighter to "stand his ground" and overcome the fear of exchanging blows with a stronger opponent. This exercise is performed by connecting two fighters with a 3-foot chain, forcing them to fight in the punching range of unarmed combat.

histrionics—The field of theatrics or acting.

hook kick—A circular kick that can be delivered in both kicking and punching ranges.

hook punch—A circular punch that can be delivered in both the punching and grappling ranges.

I

impact power—Destructive force generated by mass and velocity.

impact training—A training exercise that develops pain tolerance.

incapacitate—To disable an assailant by rendering him unconscious or damaging his bones, joints, or organs.

initiative—Making the first offensive move in combat.

inside position—The area between the opponent's arms, where he has the greatest amount of control.

intent—One of the essential factors to consider when assessing a threatening individual. The assailant's purpose or motive. See demeanor, positioning, range, and weapon capability.

intuition—The innate ability to know or sense something without the use of rational thought.

J

jersey Pull – Strategically pulling the assailant's shirt or jacket over his head as he disengages from the clinch position.

joint lock—A grappling-range technique that immobilizes the assailant's joint.

K

kick—A sudden, forceful strike with the foot.

kicking range—One of the three ranges of unarmed combat. Kicking range is the furthest distance of unarmed combat wherein you use your legs to strike an assailant. See grappling range and punching range.

kicking-range tools—The various body weapons employed in the kicking range of unarmed combat, including side kicks, push kicks, hook kicks, and vertical kicks.

killer instinct—A cold, primal mentality that surges to your consciousness and turns you into a vicious fighter.

kinesics—The study of nonlinguistic body movement communications. (For example, eye movement, shrugs, or facial gestures.)

kinesiology—The study of principles and mechanics of human movement.

kinesthetic perception—The ability to accurately feel your body during the execution of a particular movement.

knowledge—One of the three factors that determine who will win a street fight. Knowledge means knowing and understanding how to fight. See skills and attitude.

L

lead side -The side of the body that faces an assailant.

leg guard—See guard position.

linear movement—Movements that follow the path of a straight line.

low-maintenance tool—Offensive and defensive tools that require the least amount of training and practice to maintain proficiency. Low maintenance tools generally do not require preliminary stretching.

low-line kick—One of the two different classifications of a kick. A kick that is directed to targets below the assailant's waist level. (See high-line kick.)

lock—See joint lock.

M

maneuver—To manipulate into a strategically desired position.

MAP—An acronym that stands for moderate, aggressive, passive. MAP provides the practitioner with three possible responses to various grabs, chokes, and holds that occur from a standing position. See aggressive response, moderate response, and passive response.

Marathon des Sables (MdS) - a six-day, 156-mile ultramarathon held in southern Morocco, in the Sahara Desert. It is considered by many to be the toughest footrace on earth.

martial arts—The "arts of war."

masking—The process of concealing your true feelings from your opponent by manipulating and managing your body language.

mechanics—(See body mechanics.)

mental toughness - a performance mechanism utilizing a collection of mental attributes that allow a person to cope, perform and prevail through the stress of extreme adversity.

mental component—One of the three vital components of the CFA system. The mental component includes the cerebral aspects of fighting including the killer instinct, strategic and tactical development, analysis and integration, philosophy, and cognitive development. See physical component and spiritual component.

mesomorph—One of the three somatotypes. A body type classified by a high degree of muscularity and strength. The mesomorph possesses the ideal physique for unarmed combat. See ectomorph and endomorph.

mobility—A combative attribute. The ability to move your body quickly and freely while balanced. See footwork.

moderate response—One of the three possible counters when assaulted by a grab, choke, or hold from a standing position. Moderate response requires you to counter your opponent with a control and restraint (submission hold). See aggressive response and passive response.

modern martial art—A pragmatic combat art that has evolved to meet the demands and characteristics of the present time.

mounted position—A dominant ground-fighting position where a fighter straddles his opponent.

muscular endurance—The muscles' ability to perform the same

motion or task repeatedly for a prolonged period of time.

muscular flexibility—The muscles' ability to move through maximum natural ranges.

muscular strength—The maximum force that can be exerted by a particular muscle or muscle group against resistance.

muscular/skeletal conditioning—An element of physical fitness that entails muscular strength, endurance, and flexibility.

N

naked choke—A throat choke executed from the chest to back position. This secure choke is executed with two hands and it can be performed while standing, kneeling, and ground fighting with the opponent.

neck crush – A powerful pain compliance technique used when the adversary buries his head in your chest to avoid being razed.

neutralize—See incapacitate.

neutral zone—The distance outside the kicking range at which neither the practitioner nor the assailant can touch the other.

nonaggressive physiology—Strategic body language used prior to initiating a first strike.

nontelegraphic movement—Body mechanics or movements that do not inform an assailant of your intentions.

nuclear ground-fighting tools—Specific grappling range tools designed to inflict immediate and irreversible damage. Nuclear tools and tactics include biting tactics, tearing tactics, crushing tactics, continuous choking tactics, gouging techniques, raking tactics, and all striking techniques.

O

offense—The armed and unarmed means and methods of attacking a criminal assailant.

offensive flow—Continuous offensive movements (kicks, blows, and strikes) with unbroken continuity that ultimately neutralize or terminate the opponent. See compound attack.

offensive reaction time—The elapsed time between target selection and target impaction.

one-mindedness—A state of deep concentration wherein you are free from all distractions (internal and external).

ostrich defense—One of the biggest mistakes one can make when defending against an opponent. This is when the practitioner looks away from that which he fears (punches, kicks, and strikes). His mentality is, "If I can't see it, it can't hurt me."

P

pain tolerance—Your ability to physically and psychologically withstand pain.

panic—The second stage of fear; overpowering fear. See fright and terror.

parry—A defensive technique: a quick, forceful slap that redirects an assailant's linear attack. There are two types of parries: horizontal and vertical.

passive response—One of the three possible counters when assaulted by a grab, choke, or hold from a standing position. Passive response requires you to nullify the assault without injuring your adversary. See aggressive response and moderate response.

patience—A combative attribute. The ability to endure and tolerate difficulty.

perception—Interpretation of vital information acquired from your senses when faced with a potentially threatening situation.

philosophical resolution—The act of analyzing and answering various questions concerning the use of violence in defense of yourself and others.

philosophy—One of the five aspects of CFA's mental component. A deep state of introspection whereby you methodically resolve critical questions concerning the use of force in defense of yourself or others.

physical attributes—The numerous physical qualities that enhance your combative skills and abilities.

physical component—One of the three vital components of the CFA system. The physical component includes the physical aspects of fighting, such as physical fitness, weapon/technique mastery, and combative attributes. See mental component and spiritual component.

physical conditioning—See combative fitness.

physical fitness—See combative fitness.

positional asphyxia—The arrangement, placement, or positioning of your opponent's body in such a way as to interrupt your breathing and cause unconsciousness or possibly death.

positioning—The spatial relationship of the assailant to the assailed person in terms of target exposure, escape, angle of attack, and various other strategic considerations.

postal attack - see going postal.

power—A physical attribute of armed and unarmed combat. The amount of force you can generate when striking an anatomical target.

power generators—Specific points on your body that generate impact power. There are three anatomical power generators: shoulders, hips, and feet.

precision—See accuracy.

preemptive strike—See first strike.

premise—An axiom, concept, rule, or any other valid reason to modify or go beyond that which has been established.

preparedness—A state of being ready for combat. There are three components of preparedness: affective preparedness, cognitive preparedness, and psychomotor preparedness.

probable reaction dynamics - The opponent's anticipated or predicted movements or actions during both armed and unarmed combat.

proficiency training—A CFA training methodology requiring the practitioner to execute a specific body weapon, technique, maneuver, or tactic over and over for a prescribed number of repetitions. See conditioning training and street training.

proxemics—The study of the nature and effect of man's personal space.

proximity—The ability to maintain a strategically safe distance from a threatening individual.

pseudospeciation—A combative attribute. The tendency to assign subhuman and inferior qualities to a threatening assailant.

psychological conditioning—The process of conditioning the mind for the horrors and rigors of real combat.

psychomotor preparedness—One of the three components of preparedness. Psychomotor preparedness means possessing all of the physical skills and attributes necessary to defeat a formidable adversary. See affective preparedness and cognitive preparedness.

punch—A quick, forceful strike of the fists.

punching range—One of the three ranges of unarmed combat. Punching range is the mid range of unarmed combat from which the fighter uses his hands to strike his assailant. See kicking range and grappling range.

punching-range tools—The various body weapons that are employed in the punching range of unarmed combat, including finger jabs, palm-heel strikes, rear cross, knife-hand strikes, horizontal and shovel hooks, uppercuts, and hammer-fist strikes. See grappling-range tools and kicking-range tools.

Q

qualities of combat—See attributes of combat.

quarter beat - One of the four beat classifications of the Widow Maker Program. Quarter beat strikes never break contact with the assailant's face. Quarter beat strikes are primarily responsible for creating the psychological panic and trauma when Razing.

R

range—The spatial relationship between a fighter and a threatening assailant.

range deficiency—The inability to effectively fight and defend in all ranges of combat (armed and unarmed).

range manipulation—A combative attribute. The strategic manipulation of combat ranges.

range proficiency—A combative attribute. The ability to effectively fight and defend in all ranges of combat (armed and unarmed).

ranges of engagement—See combat ranges.

ranges of unarmed combat—The three distances (kicking range, punching range, and grappling range) a fighter might physically engage with an assailant while involved in unarmed combat.

raze – To level, demolish or obliterate.

razer – One who performs the Razing methodology.

razing – The second phase of the Widow Maker Program. A series of vicious close quarter techniques designed to physically and psychologically extirpate a criminal attacker.

razing amplifier - a technique, tactic or procedure that magnifies the destructiveness of your razing technique.

reaction dynamics—see probable reaction dynamics.

reaction time—The elapsed time between a stimulus and the response to that particular stimulus. See offensive reaction time and defensive reaction time.

rear cross—A straight punch delivered from the rear hand that crosses from right to left (if in a left stance) or left to right (if in a right stance).

rear side—The side of the body furthest from the assailant. See lead side.

reasonable force—That degree of force which is not excessive for a particular event and which is appropriate in protecting yourself or others.

refinement—The strategic and methodical process of improving or perfecting.

relocation principle—Also known as relocating, this is a street-fighting tactic that requires you to immediately move to a new location (usually by flanking your adversary) after delivering a compound attack.

repetition—Performing a single movement, exercise, strike, or action continuously for a specific period.

research—A scientific investigation or inquiry.

rhythm—Movements characterized by the natural ebb and flow of related elements.

ritual-oriented training—Formalized training that is conducted without intrinsic purpose. See combat-oriented training and sport-oriented training.

S

safety—One of the three criteria for a CFA body weapon, technique, maneuver, or tactic. It means that the tool, technique, maneuver or tactic provides the least amount of danger and risk for the practitioner. See efficiency and effectiveness.

scissors hold—See guard position.

scorching – Quickly and inconspicuously applying oleoresin capsicum (hot pepper extract) on your fingertips and then razing your adversary.

self-awareness—One of the three categories of CFA awareness. Knowing and understanding yourself. This includes aspects of yourself which may provoke criminal violence and which will promote a proper and strong reaction to an attack. See criminal awareness and situational awareness.

self-confidence—Having trust and faith in yourself.

self-enlightenment—The state of knowing your capabilities, limitations, character traits, feelings, general attributes, and motivations. See self-awareness.

set—A term used to describe a grouping of repetitions.

shadow fighting—A CFA training exercise used to develop and refine your tools, techniques, and attributes of armed and unarmed combat.

sharking – A counter attack technique that is used when your adversary grabs your razing hand.

shielding wedge - a defensive maneuver used to counter an unarmed postal attack.

situational awareness—One of the three categories of CFA awareness. A state of being totally alert to your immediate surroundings, including people, places, objects, and actions. (See criminal awareness and self-awareness.)

skeletal alignment—The proper alignment or arrangement of your body. Skeletal alignment maximizes the structural integrity of striking tools.

skills—One of the three factors that determine who will win a street fight. Skills refers to psychomotor proficiency with the tools and techniques of combat. See Attitude and Knowledge.

slipping—A defensive maneuver that permits you to avoid an assailant's linear blow without stepping out of range. Slipping can be accomplished by quickly snapping the head and upper torso sideways (right or left) to avoid the blow.

snap back—A defensive maneuver that permits you to avoid an assailant's linear and circular blows without stepping out of range. The snap back can be accomplished by quickly snapping the head backward to avoid the assailant's blow.

somatotypes—A method of classifying human body types or builds into three different categories: endomorph, mesomorph, and ectomorph. See endomorph, mesomorph, and ectomorph.

sparring—A training exercise where two or more fighters fight each other while wearing protective equipment.

speed—A physical attribute of armed and unarmed combat. The rate or a measure of the rapid rate of motion.

spiritual component—One of the three vital components of the CFA system. The spiritual component includes the metaphysical issues and aspects of existence. See physical component and mental component.

sport-oriented training—Training that is geared for competition and governed by a set of rules. See combat-oriented training and ritual-oriented training.

sprawling—A grappling technique used to counter a double- or single-leg takedown.

square off—To be face-to-face with a hostile or threatening assailant who is about to attack you.

stance—One of the many strategic postures you assume prior to or during armed or unarmed combat.

stick fighting—Fighting that takes place with either one or two sticks.

strategic positioning—Tactically positioning yourself to either escape, move behind a barrier, or use a makeshift weapon.

strategic/tactical development—One of the five elements of CFA's mental component.

strategy—A carefully planned method of achieving your goal of engaging an assailant under advantageous conditions.

street fight—A spontaneous and violent confrontation between two or more individuals wherein no rules apply.

street fighter—An unorthodox combatant who has no formal training. His combative skills and tactics are usually developed in the street by the process of trial and error.

street training—A CFA training methodology requiring the practitioner to deliver explosive compound attacks for 10 to 20 seconds. See condition ng training and proficiency training.

strength training—The process of developing muscular strength through systematic application of progressive resistance.

stress - physiological and psychological arousal caused by a stressor.

stressors - any activity, situation, circumstance, event, experience, or condition that causes a person to experience both physiological and psychological stress.

striking art—A combat art that relies predominantly on striking techniques to neutralize or terminate a criminal attacker.

striking shield—A rectangular shield constructed of foam and vinyl used to develop power in your kicks, punches, and strikes.

striking tool—A natural body weapon that impacts with the assailant's anatomical target.

strong side—The strongest and most coordinated side of your body.

structure—A definite and organized pattern.

style—The distinct manner in which a fighter executes or performs his combat skills.

stylistic integration—The purposeful and scientific collection of tools and techniques from various disciplines, which are strategically integrated and dramatically altered to meet three essential criteria: efficiency, effectiveness, and combative safety.

submission holds—Also known as control and restraint techniques, many of these locks and holds create sufficient pain to cause the adversary to submit.

system—The unification of principles, philosophies, rules, strategies, methodologies, tools, and techniques of a particular method of combat.

T

tactic—The skill of using the available means to achieve an end.

target awareness—A combative attribute that encompasses five strategic principles: target orientation, target recognition, target selection, target impaction, and target exploitation.

target exploitation—A combative attribute. The strategic maximization of your assailant's reaction dynamics during a fight. Target exploitation can be applied in both armed and unarmed encounters.

target impaction—The successful striking of the appropriate anatomical target.

target orientation—A combative attribute. Having a workable knowledge of the assailant's anatomical targets.

target recognition—The ability to immediately recognize appropriate anatomical targets during an emergency self-defense situation.

target selection—The process of mentally selecting the appropriate anatomical target for your self-defense situation. This is predicated on certain factors, including proper force response, assailant's positioning, and range.

target stare—A form of telegraphing in which you stare at the anatomical target you intend to strike.

target zones—The three areas in which an assailant's anatomical targets are located. (See zone one, zone two and zone three.)

technique—A systematic procedure by which a task is accomplished.

telegraphic cognizance—A combative attribute. The ability to recognize both verbal and non-verbal signs of aggression or assault.

telegraphing—Unintentionally making your intentions known to your adversary.

tempo—The speed or rate at which you speak.

terminate—To kill.

terror—The third stage of fear; defined as overpowering fear. See fright and panic.

timing—A physical and mental attribute of armed and unarmed combat. Your ability to execute a movement at the optimum moment.

tone—The overall quality or character of your voice.

tool—See body weapon.

traditional martial arts—Any martial art that fails to evolve and change to meet the demands and characteristics of its present environment.

traditional style/system—See traditional martial arts.

training drills—The various exercises and drills aimed at perfecting combat skills, attributes, and tactics.

trap and tuck – A counter move technique used when the adversary attempts to raze you during your quarter beat assault.

U

unified mind—A mind free and clear of distractions and focused on the combative situation.

use of force response—A combative attribute. Selecting the appropriate level of force for a particular emergency self-defense situation.

V

viciousness—A combative attribute. The propensity to be extremely violent and destructive often characterized by intense savagery.

violence—The intentional utilization of physical force to coerce, injure, cripple, or kill.

visualization—Also known as mental visualization or mental imagery. The purposeful formation of mental images and scenarios in the mind's eye.

W

warm-up—A series of mild exercises, stretches, and movements designed to prepare you for more intense exercise.

weak side—The weaker and more uncoordinated side of your body.

weapon and technique mastery—A component of CFA's physical component. The kinesthetic and psychomotor development of a weapon or combative technique.

weapon capability—An assailant's ability to use and attack with a particular weapon.

webbing - The first phase of the Widow Maker Program. Webbing is a two hand strike delivered to the assailant's chin. It is called Webbing because your hands resemble a large web that wraps around the enemy's face.

widow maker – One who makes widows by destroying husbands.

widow maker program – A CFA combat program specifically designed to teach the law abiding citizen how to use extreme force when faced with immediate threat of unlawful deadly criminal attack. The Widow Maker program is divided into two phases or methodologies: Webbing and Razing.

Y

yell—A loud and aggressive scream or shout used for various strategic reasons.

Z

zero beat – One of the four beat classifications of the Widow Maker, Feral Fighting and Savage Street Fighting Programs. Zero beat strikes are full pressure techniques applied to a specific target until it completely ruptures. They include gouging, crushing, biting, and choking techniques.

zone one—Anatomical targets related to your senses, including the eyes, temple, nose, chin, and back of neck.

zone three—Anatomical targets related to your mobility, including thighs, knees, shins, and instep.

zone two—Anatomical targets related to your breathing, including front of neck, solar plexus, ribs, and groin.

Cane Fighting

About Sammy Franco

With over 30 years of experience, Sammy Franco is one of the world's foremost authorities on armed and unarmed self-defense. Highly regarded as a leading innovator in martial arts, Mr. Franco was one of the premier pioneers in the field of "reality-based" self-defense and combat instruction.

Sammy Franco is perhaps best known as the founder and creator of Contemporary Fighting Arts (CFA), a state-of-the-art offensive-based combat system that is specifically designed for real-world self-defense. CFA is a sophisticated and practical system of self-defense, designed specifically to provide efficient and effective methods to avoid, defuse, confront, and neutralize both armed and unarmed attackers.

Sammy Franco has frequently been featured in martial art magazines, newspapers, and appeared on numerous radio and television programs. Mr. Franco has also authored numerous books, magazine articles, and editorials and has developed a popular library of instructional videos.

Sammy Franco's experience and credibility in the combat science is unequaled. One of his many accomplishments in this field includes the fact that he has earned the ranking of a Law Enforcement Master Instructor, and has designed, implemented, and taught officer survival training to the United States Border Patrol (USBP). He has instructed members of the US Secret Service, Military Special Forces, Washington DC Police Department, Montgomery County, Maryland

Cane Fighting

Deputy Sheriffs, and the US Library of Congress Police. Sammy Franco is also a member of the prestigious International Law Enforcement Educators and Trainers Association (ILEETA) as well as the American Society of Law Enforcement Trainers (ASLET) and he is listed in the "Who's Who Director of Law Enforcement Instructors."

Sammy Franco is also a nationally certified Law Enforcement Instructor in the following curricula: PR-24 Side-Handle Baton, Police Arrest and Control Procedures, Police Personal Weapons Tactics, Police Power Handcuffing Methods, Police Oleoresin Capsicum Aerosol Training (OCAT), Police Weapon Retention and Disarming Methods, Police Edged Weapon Countermeasures and "Use of Force" Assessment and Response Methods.

Mr. Franco regularly conducts dynamic and enlightening seminars on different aspects of combat training, mental toughness and achieving personal peak performance.

On a personal level, Sammy Franco is an animal lover, who will go to great lengths to assist and rescue animals. Throughout the years, he's rescued everything from turkey vultures to goats. However, his most treasured moments are always spent with his beloved German Shepherd dogs.

For more information about Mr. Franco, you can visit his website at **SammyFranco.com** or follow him on Twitter **@RealSammyFranco**

Other Books by Sammy Franco

KUBOTAN POWER
Quick and Simple Steps to Mastering the Kubotan Keychain
by Sammy Franco

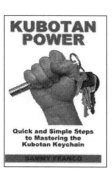

With over 290 photographs and step-by-step instructions, Kubotan Power is the authoritative resource for mastering this devastating self-defense weapon. In this one-of-a-kind book, world-renowned self-defense expert, Sammy Franco takes thirty years of real-world teaching experience and gives you quick, easy and practical kubotan techniques that can be used by civilians, law enforcement personnel, or military professionals. 8.5 x 5.5, paperback, 290 photos, illustrations, 204 pages.

FIRST STRIKE
End a Fight in Ten Seconds or Less!
by Sammy Franco

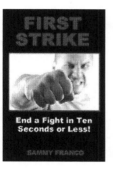

Learn how to stop any attack before it starts by mastering the art of the preemptive strike. First Strike gives you an easy-to-learn yet highly effective self-defense game plan for handling violent close-quarter combat encounters. First Strike will teach you instinctive, practical and realistic self-defense techniques that will drop any criminal attacker to the floor with one punishing blow. By reading this book and by practicing, you will learn the hard-hitting skills necessary to execute a punishing first strike and ultimately prevail in a self-defense situation. 8.5 x 5.5, paperback, photos, illustrations, 202 pages.

MAXIMUM DAMAGE
Hidden Secrets Behind Brutal Fighting Combination
by Sammy Franco

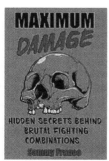

Maximum Damage teaches you the quickest ways to beat your opponent by exploiting his physical and psychological reactions in a fight. Learn how to stay two steps ahead of your adversary by knowing exactly how he will react to your strikes before they are delivered. In this unique book, self-defense expert Sammy Franco reveals his unique Probable Reaction Dynamic (PRD) fighting method. Probable reaction dynamics are both a scientific and comprehensive offensive strategy based on the positional theory of combat. Regardless of your style of fighting, PRD training will help you overpower your opponent by integrating your strikes into brutal fighting combinations that are fast, ferocious and final! 8.5 x 5.5, paperback, 240 photos, illustrations, 238 pages.

HEAVY BAG TRAINING
For Boxing, Mixed Martial Arts and Self-Defense
(Heavy Bag Training Series Book 1)

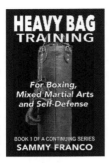

by Sammy Franco

The heavy bag is one of the oldest and most recognizable pieces of training equipment. It's used by boxers, mixed martial artists, self-defense practitioners, and fitness enthusiasts. Unfortunately, most people don't know how to use the heavy bag correctly. Heavy Bag Training teaches you everything you ever wanted to know about working out on the heavy bag. In this one-of-a-kind book, world-renowned self-defense expert Sammy Franco provides you with the knowledge, skills, and attitude necessary to maximize the training benefits of the bag. 8.5 x 5.5, paperback, photos, illus, 172 pages.

HEAVY BAG COMBINATIONS
The Ultimate Guide to Heavy Bag Punching Combinations
(Heavy Bag Training Series Book 2)

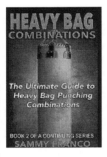

by Sammy Franco

Heavy Bag Combinations is the second book in Sammy Franco's best-selling Heavy Bag Training Series. This unique book is your ultimate guide to mastering devastating heavy bag punching combinations. With over 300+ photographs and detailed step-by-step instructions, Heavy Bag Combinations provides beginner, intermediate and advanced heavy bag workout combinations that will challenge you for the rest of your life! In fact, even the most experienced athlete will advance his fighting skills to the next level and beyond. 8.5 x 5.5, paperback, photos, illus, 248 pages.

THE COMPLETE BODY OPPONENT BAG BOOK

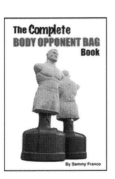

by Sammy Franco

In this one-of-a-kind book, Sammy Franco teaches you the many hidden training features of the body opponent bag that will improve your fighting skills and boost your conditioning. With detailed photographs, step-by-step instructions, and dozens of unique workout routines, The Complete Body Opponent Bag Book is the authoritative resource for mastering this lifelike punching bag. It covers stances, punching, kicking, grappling techniques, mobility and footwork, targets, fighting ranges, training gear, time based workouts, punching and kicking combinations, weapons training, grappling drills, ground fighting, and dozens of workouts. 8.5 x 5.5, paperback, 139 photos, illustrations, 206 pages.

INVINCIBLE
Mental Toughness Techniques for the Street, Battlefield and Playing Field
by Sammy Franco

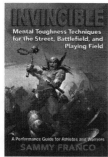

Invincible is a treasure trove of battle-tested techniques and strategies for improving mental toughness in all aspects of life. It teaches you how to unlock the true power of your mind and achieve success in sports, fitness, high-risk professions, self-defense, and other peak performance activities. However, you don't have to be an athlete or warrior to benefit from this unique mental toughness book. In fact, the mental skills featured in this indispensable program can be used by anyone who wants to reach their full potential in life. 8.5 x 5.5, paperback, photos, illus, 250 pages.

THE WIDOW MAKER PROGRAM
Extreme Self-Defense for Deadly Force Situations
by Sammy Franco

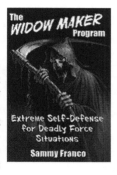

The Widow Maker Program is a shocking and revolutionary fighting style designed to unleash extreme force when faced with the immediate threat of an unlawful deadly criminal attack. In this unique book, self-defense innovator Sammy Franco teaches you his brutal and unorthodox combat style that is virtually indefensible and utterly devastating. With over 250 photographs and detailed step-by-step instructions, The Widow Maker Program teaches you Franco's surreptitious Webbing and Razing techniques. When combined, these two fighting methods create an unstoppable force capable of destroying the toughest adversary. 8.5 x 5.5, paperback, photos, illus, 218 pages.

FERAL FIGHTING
Advanced Widow Maker Fighting Techniques
by Sammy Franco

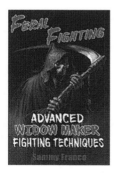

In this sequel, Sammy Franco marches forward with cutting-edge concepts and techniques that will take your self-defense skills to entirely new levels of combat performance. Feral Fighting includes Franco's revolutionary Shielding Wedge technique. When used correctly, it transforms you into an unstoppable human meat grinder, capable of destroying any criminal adversary. Feral Fighting also teaches you the cunning art or Scorching. Learn how to convert your fingertips into burning torches that generate over 2 million scoville heat units causing excruciating pain and temporarily blindness. 8.5 x 5.5, paperback, photos, illustrations, 204 pages.

SAVAGE STREET FIGHTING
Tactical Savagery as a Last Resort
by Sammy Franco

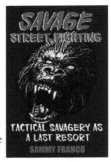

In this revolutionary book, Sammy Franco reveals the science behind his most primal street fighting method. Savage Street Fighting is a brutal self-defense system specifically designed to teach the law-abiding citizen how to use "Tactical Savagery" when faced with the immediate threat of an unlawful deadly criminal attack. Savage Street Fighting is systematically engineered to protect you when there are no other self-defense options left! With over 300 photographs and detailed step-by-step instructions, Savage Street Fighting is a must-have book for anyone concerned about real world self-defense. Now is the time to learn how to unleash your inner beast! 8.5 x 5.5, paperback, 317 photos, illustrations, 232 pages.

WAR MACHINE
How to Transform Yourself Into A Vicious & Deadly Street Fighter
by Sammy Franco

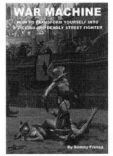

War Machine is a book that will change you for the rest of your life! When followed accordingly, War Machine will forge your mind, body and spirit into iron. Once armed with the mental and physical attributes of the War Machine, you will become a strong and confident warrior that can handle just about anything that life may throw your way. In essence, War Machine is a way of life. Powerful, intense, and hard. 11 x 8.5, paperback, photos, illustrations, 210 pages.

CONTEMPORARY FIGHTING ARTS, LLC
"Real World Self-Defense Since 1989"
SammyFranco.com